How to See Like a Hawk When You're Blind as a Bat

A Patient's Guide to LASIK Laser Vision Correction

Matthew Ehrlich, M.D.

Published by
Doctor's Advice Press
217 the Esplanade South
Venice, FL 34285
www.lasikbook.com

Publisher's Cataloging-in-Publication Data

Ehrlich, Matthew

  How to see like a hawk when you're blind
as a bat : a patient's guide to LASIK laser
vision correction / Matthew Ehrlich. —
Venice, FL : Doctors Advice Press, 1999.

    p. cm.
Includes index
ISBN: 0-9669272-0-6

  1. Cornea — Laser surgery — Popular works.
I. Title.

RE336 .E47 1999   99-61193
617 . 7/55 — dc21   CIP

Printed in the United States of America
10 9 8 7 6 5 4 3 2

Dedication

To Diane, whose love supported me through this journey.

Acknowledgments

I would like to thank my colleagues who reviewed the manuscript: Richard Abbott, M.D., Stephen Brint, M.D., and Richard Lindstrom, M.D. Carolyn Porter and Alan Gadney spent many hours in the editing and production of the book. George Foster brought the cover to life, and David Utz the graphic illustrations. I would also like to thank my professors at Wills Eye Hospital and the Jules Stein Eye Institute at UCLA, especially Lee Nordan, M.D., and the thousands of patients who have made my career in laser vision correction possible.

About the Medical Reviewers of this Book:

Richard Abbott, M.D. is professor of ophthalmology at the University of California at San Francisco, and co-director of the UCSF Beckman Vision Center. He served on the FDA committee that approved PRK in 1995 and participated in the FDA clinical trials on intrastromal corneal ring segments.

Stephen Brint, M.D. served as clinical investigator for Summit laser for the FDA trials and remains an active investigator. He travels the world in pursuit of new techniques and performed the first LASIK procedure in the U.S. in 1991. Steve is often called upon to demonstrate live surgery via satellite to major ophthalmology conferences.

Richard Lindstrom, M.D., clinical professor of ophthalmology at the University of Minnesota, practiced full time at the university before returning to private practice. While chairman of the ophthalmology department his corneal fellowship training program was one of the most sought after in the country. Dr. Lindstrom is often invited to lecture at major ophthalmology meetings. He was a clinical investigator of PRK for the VISX, FDA trials and remains an active clinical investigator for VISX.

Foreword

Informed consent is the ethical basis of the practice of medicine. Unfortunately, over the years there has been a lot more consenting than informing. The problem is that informed consent is much more than a patient merely signing his or her name at the bottom of a form whose print requires a magnifier to read. To function properly informed consent must be an active, educational process on the part of both the doctor and the patient which ultimately permits a knowledgeable decision to be made by the patient whether the benefits of a medical procedure or treatment outweigh the possible risks. This can be a difficult decision, particularly for an elective procedure that involves precious eyesight on healthy eyes.

The debate about the pros and cons of refractive surgery in general and LASIK in particular is a case in point. Getting information is not easy. Sources tend to be either too simple or biased (waiting room pamphlets and commercially prepared videos), or too complicated (professional treatises). Internet sites contain some information but it is mostly promotional or anecdotal. Direct discussions between the doctor and the patient are frequently influenced by time constraints.

Dr. Matthew Ehrlich has made an honest attempt to fill the void in relation to LASIK Laser Vision Correction in the following book. I personally believe that it should be read by anyone contemplating this procedure or refractive surgery in general.

Robin Cook

Contents

Introduction:
What is Laser Vision Correction?

*D*oes any of this sound familiar?

- You fumble for your eyeglasses on the nightstand before attempting to get out of bed.

- Your glasses fog as you get out of your car or venture in and out of a few stores to shop.

- Your eyes are red, dry and irritated from your contact lenses, and you've got hours before you can get home to take them out. To make matters worse, your vision's getting blurry.

- You never can clearly see:

  - The hair in the shower, let alone your feet.

  - The sight of your lover in bed.

  - The road ahead as you jog down the street in the rain, removing your glasses to wipe them as you run—those damn glasses that keep slipping down your nose as you perspire.

- You forgot to pack your contact lens disinfecting solution and there's not a drug store open for a hundred miles.

- Your hand smacks into the wall of the swimming pool or the man swimming just ahead that you just did not see.

"What, are you blind!" he shouts at you.

In fact, millions of Americans have vision equivalent to legal blindness when they are not their wearing glasses or contact lenses.

This is what the miracle of laser vision correction is all about, allowing people to function without the disability of requiring corrective lenses.

Only a person who must rely on his glasses to see can truly understand the handicap from which he suffers. If that person is you or a loved one, keep reading. The purpose of this book is to answer your questions about this exciting new laser surgery. You will learn if you are a candidate, how successful the procedure is, what the possible complications are, and if there is something better on the horizon.

Laser Vision Correction Is Not a Cure for Eye Diseases

Laser vision correction is not a means of correcting eye diseases such as lazy eye or amblyopia, crossed eyes, macular degeneration or other retinal disorders. It will not allow you, except in extreme cases of nearsightedness, to see more sharply than you do with your contact lenses or glasses. It does not eliminate the need for reading glasses. In fact, if you are near the age of forty and need glasses for seeing in the distance, but not for reading, the reverse may occur after laser surgery. More on that later.

Refractive Surgery Has Never Been Better

Refractive surgery has been my passion since my fellowship at the Jules Stein Eye Institute, University of California at Los Angeles (UCLA) in 1987-1988. At that time radial keratotomy was our primary modality of treatment. Lamellar procedures—where a layer of the cornea was cut with a special machine, frozen, then carved into a human contact lens and sewn back on the eye—were in limited use for extremely myopic patients. Results back then were encouraging in well-trained hands but pale in comparison with the computerized excimer laser now available.

In my ten years in this field, I have never been more excited than now about what we can offer you. Join me in this quest. *Read on.*

Disclaimer

A sincere effort has been made to present the risks and benefits of laser vision correction. The opinions expressed are those of the author. Before deciding to undergo laser vision correction, LASIK or PRK, you must consult with the surgeon who is performing the procedure. You need to know for your specific case, and in your surgeon's hands what the risks are to you and the probability of achieving the vision you desire.

1
Are You a Candidate?

Your next logical question is whether or not you're a candidate for laser vision correction. In order to answer this, we first need to define some terms and explain how the eye focuses light.

A person who needs glasses or contact lenses to see has a "**refractive error**." There are four types of refractive errors:

- myopia or nearsightedness

- hyperopia or farsightedness

- astigmatism

- presbyopia

Any type of surgery to correct one of these conditions—radial keratotomy, excimer laser, corneal rings or intraocular lenses—is called "**refractive surgery**." A person whose eyesight is perfect and lacks any of the above four conditions is "**emmetropic**." It is common to have more than one type of refractive error. Myopic (near-sighted) patients often have astigmatism and/or pres-byopia, as do hyperopic (farsighted) patients.

How Does the Eye Focus Light?

The eye has two lenses that focus light on its back surface, or retina (figure 1). These are the cornea and the crystalline lens. The cornea is the clear outer window. When we look into someone's eyes we fail to notice the transparent cornea, but instead observe the color of the iris—brown, blue, or green—inside his eye. If you have a pet at home, look at its eye from the side to appreciate the clear dome of the cornea.

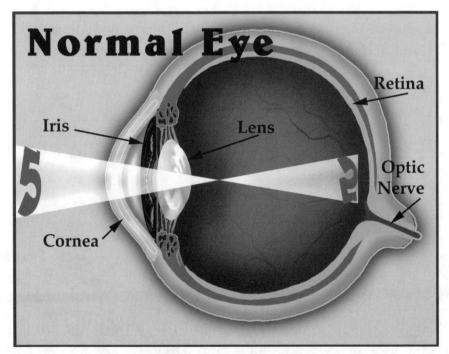

Figure 1 — Normal eye

The path of light through the eye begins at the cornea, continues across the fluid filled anterior chamber, through the pupil or round opening of the iris, through the **crystalline lens**, across the large vitreous jelly cavity, and finally is focused on the retina. While the cornea cannot change its focus, the crystalline lens can adjust its power, a process known as "accommodation." The lens of the eye is familiar to us from the term "**cataract**," which is a cloudiness that occurs due to age (figure 2).

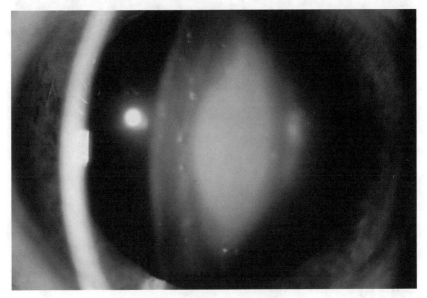

Figure 2 — Cataract

There are several ways to correct the focus of an eye that needs eyeglasses. These will be explored in chapter six. However, all refractive surgery utilizes one of two means to accomplish its goal. One is by changing the curvature of the cornea, the other is by replacing the crystalline lens, or modifying its power with the insertion of an additional lens. We routinely modify refractive error in patients with cataracts by replacing their clouded lens with a plastic one, known as an "implant" or "**intraocular lens**" (see figure 3). Modification of the corneal power by laser is the main topic of this book and a key method to correct refractive errors since 66 percent of the focusing power of the eye comes from the cornea and 34 percent from the adjustable crystalline lens.

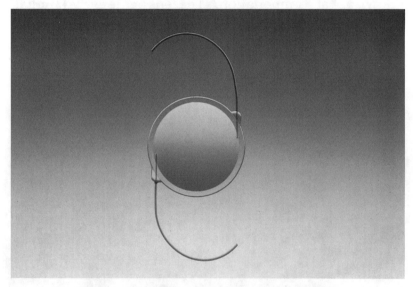

Figure 3 —Implant or "intraocular lens"
Courtesy of Bausch & Lomb Surgical

The Eye Can Alter its Focus

The normal eye has the ability to increase or relax its focusing power, similar to an autofocusing lens in a camera. Of the two lenses mentioned above, only the crystalline lens can do this. "**Accommodation**" is the process by which we change our focus from a distant object to a near one, as when we read. The lens accomplishes this by changing its shape and needs to be elastic to do this. Two other actions happen to our eyes as we accommodate: 1. our pupils become smaller, and 2. our eyes converge inwards. When we change our focus from a near point to a distant one, as when we look up from reading to focus on trees outside our window, we "relax our accommodation." Our pupils dilate, our eyes diverge, and our lenses change their shape.

Children have incredible powers of accommodation, measuring sixteen units or more at age five. In contrast, by the time we are forty our accommodative power has reduced to 4.5 units, and by the time we are sixty-five, 0.75 units.

Drugs which block accommodation are called "**cycloplegic agents**." As a patient, you have experienced these as "**dilating drops**" that blur your vision, making it difficult to read. These drops make it easier to see inside your eye because they dilate your pupil.

Refractive Errors—Reasons Why People Need Eyeglasses to See

1. Presbyopia

Over the years our lenses progressively lose their elasticity and the ability to accommodate. We refer to this as "**presbyopia**" or "old sight." For most people this becomes noticeable in their early to mid-forties. They usually complain that they have to hold the newspaper farther away in order to read it. This is the time to begin using reading glasses or bifocals. Presbyopia worsens with age making stronger corrective lenses necessary.

Even people who have had perfect eyesight before forty develop presbyopia, just as do those whose vision has been poor for other reasons (see below). It's simply part of getting older. Laser vision correction does not yet offer any direct treatment for presbyopia. However, an indirect treatment consists of correcting one eye for far vision and one eye for near, a situation known as "**monovision**."

2. Myopia or Nearsightedness

If the lenses of the eye, cornea and/or crystalline lens, are too powerful, they will focus an image in front of the retina instead of directly on it. Alternatively, if the lenses have a normal amount of power but the eye grows too long, the same situation will occur (figure 4). This explains why children with myopia need progressively stronger glasses as they mature. The length of their eyes continues to grow and the images become farther out of focus. Only one millimeter of extra length will create three diopters of myopia (see pg.17 for explanation of diopters). People with myopia, or "**myopes**," will often begin wearing glasses in elementary school and progress until stabilizing in their mid to late twenties. In later years myopia can increase again with cataract development.

Myopes are divided into low, moderate, and high categories based on the strength of their eyeglass lenses. **Low myopia** refers to patients needing up to three diopters of correction, **moderate myopia** from three to six diopters, and **high myopia** greater than six diopters.

Myopes cannot see clearly in the distance and their crystalline lens cannot adjust the focus for them. In other words, accommodation would make their distance vision worse. The best they can do to attempt to see in the distance is to fully relax their accommodation, but even this is not enough for a myope. They can, however, focus on objects that are near. Thus the expression "**nearsighted**" arose for these patients. As they become presbyopic, many patients with low myopia will remove their glasses to read.

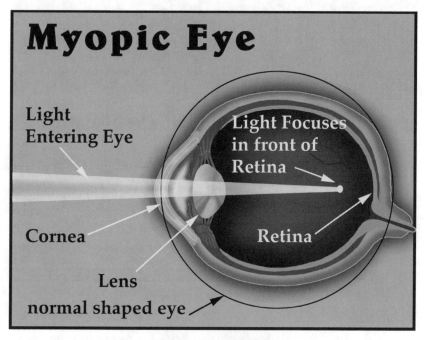

Myopic Eye

Light
Entering Eye

Light Focuses
in front of
Retina

Cornea

Retina

Lens

normal shaped eye

Figure 4 — Myopia

In contrast, the near vision of moderate to high myopes is of limited utility. Their prescription is so strong that their near focus is only inches in front of their noses and they will usually use reading glasses. Therefore, in electing to undergo laser vision correction, losing near vision without glasses for moderate to high myopes is not nearly as important an issue as gaining distance vision. Most will happily make this compromise.

3. Hyperopia or Farsightedness

If the combined power of the cornea and crystalline lens is too weak, images will remain unfocused and pass through the retina or behind the eye (figure 5A).

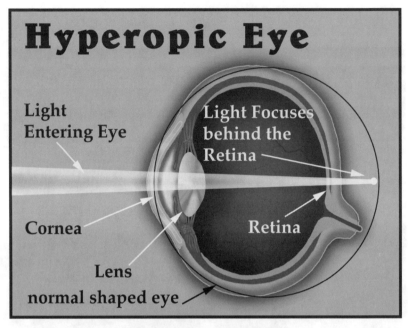

Figure 5A — Hyperopia

Alternatively, if the power of the lenses is normal but the eye is abnormally short in its length, the same focusing error arises. Unlike myopes, "**hyperopes**" can, to a degree, overcome their refractive error and focus by accommodating (figure 5B). Depending on the amount of hyperopia, they may be able to focus without glasses. As the amount of hyperopia increases, however, they begin to have trouble. Since it takes more accommodative power to focus at near than at a distance, the first problem will manifest when reading. Typically these people experience eye strain or headaches. Their distance vision may be a perfect 20/20, but reading vision is difficult. This leads to the term "farsightedness" to describe hyperopes. It is, however, a misleading term. As the degree of hyperopia progresses, the person will no longer be able to focus in the distance either. Thus, people with higher levels of hyperopia cannot see clearly at far or near, and they do not understand why they are described as **"farsighted."**

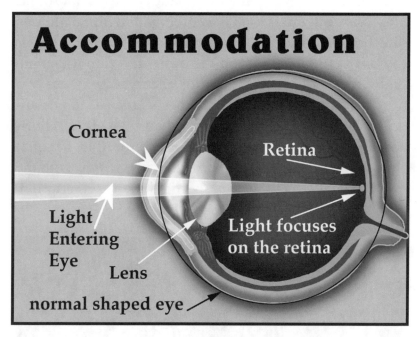

Figure 5B — Accommodation

You may notice some children who wear extremely strong magnifying eyeglasses and whose eyes turn in without them. This is a type of "crossed eyes" problem called accommodative esotropia. They are so hyperopic that when they struggle to focus on a distant object they maximize their accommodation and their eyes turn inward too much as a result. As you recall, part of the accommodative response is for the eyes to turn inward (see pg.4). When children are given glasses to correct their hyperopia, they relax their accommodation and their eyes straighten. Hyperopia also increases with age, as the ability to "accommodate" or focus the eye is progressively lost.

4. Astigmatism

The Latin derivation of **astigmatism** is "a" for not, and "stigmata" for round. The astigmatic cornea is not round like a baseball but is oval like a football (figure 6). In one direction the cornea is curved more steeply with a shorter radius of curvature, and in the other direction it is more flatly curved with a longer radius of curvature. These two directions or "**axes**" are usually perpendicular to one another. Typically one axis is vertical and the other is horizontal (figure 7). Eyeglasses correct for this unequal curvature by putting more correction in one axis, with the exact orientation of this axis specified in the prescription, such as 90 degrees, 180 degrees, 45 degrees, etc.

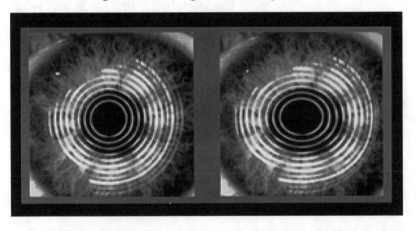

A. Normal eye   B. Astigmatic eye

Figure 6—Astigmatic cornea
Courtesy American Academy of Ophthalmology

Most patients have **regular astigmatism**. Although the surface of their cornea is not round it is smooth. Their astigmatism is readily correctable by eyeglasses or contact lenses. Occasionally a patient has an **irregular astigma-**

tism. The surface of his cornea is not round and also not smooth. Irregular astigmatism cannot be fully corrected by glasses. It requires a semi-rigid, gas permeable contact lens that presents a smooth outer surface to the world.

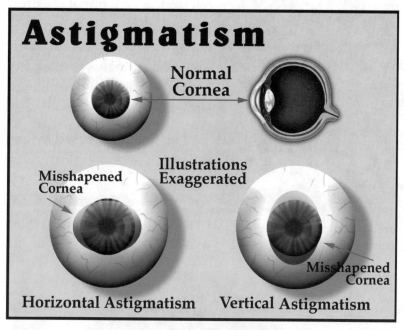

Astigmatism

Normal Cornea

Illustrations Exaggerated

Misshapened Cornea

Misshapened Cornea

Horizontal Astigmatism   Vertical Astigmatism

Figure 7 — Astigmatism

Corneal topography has done much to help us understand astigmatism by showing us a map of the surface of the eye. A special machine begins by taking a video image of a series of illuminated rings projected onto a patient's cornea (figures 6 and 8). The information is then fed into a computer that can produce a colored map of the contour of the entire corneal surface. Using the colors of the rainbow, more steep areas of curvature are shown in darker colors, and flat areas appear lighter (figure 9).

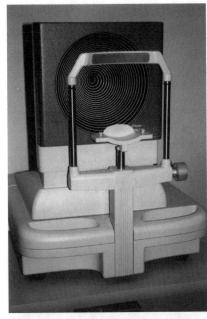

Figure 8—Corneal Topographer
Courtesy of Alcon Surgical

To further complicate matters, some patients have a spherical cornea but an astigmatic crystalline lens. This is referred to as **lenticular astigmatism**. The patient's eyeglasses correct for the net astigmatism that is created by both corneal and crystalline lenses.

The images focused by an astigmatic eye are blurred at both near and far focus. At any one time the image of an object will be in focus in one axis but not the other— hori-

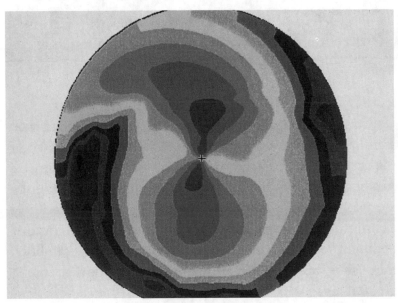

Figure 9—Corneal map demonstrating a vertically steep cornea

zontally, but not vertically, for example. The crystalline lens cannot correct this refractive error by accommodation. It would bring both axes to a closer focus in the eye but one would remain out of focus in relation to the other. For this reason, astigmatism distorts both distance as well as near vision. The greater the astigmatism the greater the distortion. Most people have some astigmatism, but for most it is mild enough to cause no noticeable problem.

As will be discussed later, the excimer laser can treat this unequal curvature of the cornea with good accuracy.

How Can You Tell What Type of Refractive Error You Have?

The easiest way to determine your refractive error is to look at a copy of your eyeglass or contact lens prescription (figure 10). There are generally four columns: sphere, cylinder or power of astigmatism, axis of astigmatism, and prism. The first line on the prescription is for **O.D.**, or **ocular dexter** (the right eye), and the next line for **O.S.**, **ocular sinister** (the left eye). (Note the societal bias against left handedness!)

In the first column, the sphere, you will find out if you are a myope or a hyperope. Myopes have a minus sign in this column and hyperopes a plus sign. The number following the plus or minus sign shows the power or degree of myopia or hyperopia. The higher the number the stronger the prescription. Increments of 0.25 are used. A common term for zero, or no spherical error, is "**plano.**"

In the second column the strength of the astigmatism or cylinder is shown, also in 0.25 increments. The minus or plus sign preceeding the astigmatism power in the second column has nothing to do with myopia or hyperopia: just ignore it.

		SPH	CYL	AXIS	PRISM
Distance	OD				
	OS				
Add	OD				
	OS				

Figure 10 —Eyeglass prescription form

The third column shows the axis of the astigmatism that is being corrected. If there is nothing in the second or third columns then you have no astigmatism. Your prescription is spherical. The fourth column, prism, is for patients with crossed eyes or other misalignment of the eye muscles. Contact lens bottles will have the same information printed on them, except for prism.

If you have no presciption or contact lens bottle to review, you can get some insight from your eyeglasses. If your eyes look smaller or minimized (i.e., "beady eyed") with your glasses on, you are a myope. It is common to see reflections or rings in the outer edge of your glasses (figure 11). Compare this to looking through the bottom of a coke bottle. A myope's glasses are thicker at the edges than in the center. For cosmetic reasons, moderate to high myopes should select smaller eyeglass frame sizes to minimize the thickness of the lenses.

In contrast, a hyperope's eyes look magnified through their glasses. The center of their lenses are thicker than the periphery.

Astigmatism is harder to appreciate from a visual inspection of your eyeglasses. Hold them a few inches in front of your eyes while you view a distant object. Now rotate the stems of the glasses and see if the image you are watching appears to distort. Because an astigmatic eyeglass lens has varying power in different axes, the image will change as you rotate the glasses.

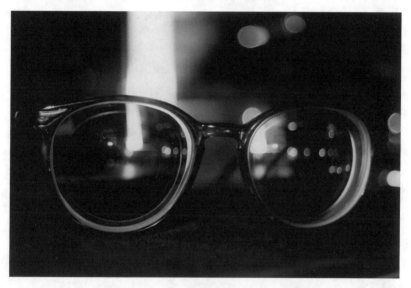

Figure 11—Eyeglasses for myopia

All of these observations depend upon the strength of an individual's prescription. The stronger the correction the more obvious the above descriptions will be. Minimal prescriptions may be difficult to observe.

How Does Laser Corneal Refractive Surgery Work?

This type of surgery changes the power of the corneal lens—it's that simple.

To correct myopia the laser flattens the corneal curvature to reduce its focusing strength. The laser thins the center of the cornea by vaporizing a small amount of tissue, which is of lesser thickness than a human hair. More will be said about this later.

To correct hyperopia the laser steepens the central corneal curvature, which increases the power of the corneal lens. The laser accomplishes this by flattening the periphery of the cornea, allowing the central cornea to protrude or steepen.

For astigmatism correction the axis with the steep curvature can be flattened or the flat axis steepened to create a spherical or round corneal curvature. The treatment is oval shaped applying excimer laser to both perpendicular axes but more to one axis than another (figure 12).

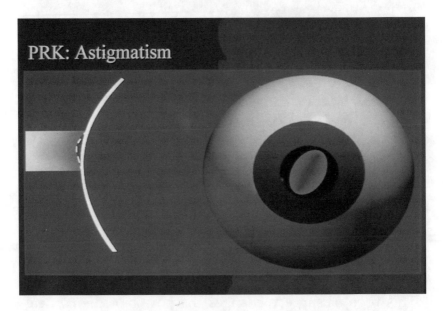

Figure 12—Laser Correction of Astigmatism
Courtesy of VISX

The Strength of Your Refractive Error

Measuring anything require standard units. To measure weight we use pounds in the U.S., kilograms in Europe.

For refractive errors, eyeglass lenses and contact lenses, the units are known as "**diopters.**" A one diopter lens is one that can bring rays of light into focus 1 meter (about 3 feet) behind the lens (figure 13). A two diopter lens is twice as strong and will bring the same rays of light to a focus a half a meter from the lens. A five diopter lens has a focal length of one-fifth of a meter, or less than a foot.

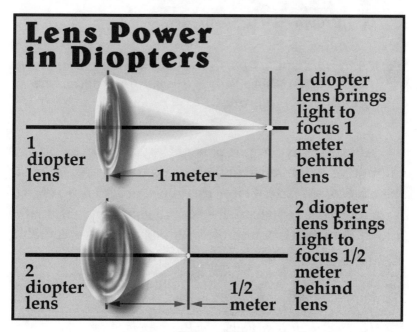

Figure 13

Enough Already—Am I a Candidate or Not?

FDA approval is granted to individual laser manufacturers as they submit their results. Thus, one laser may be approved to treat higher degrees of myopia, hyperopia, or astigmatism than another.

In the U.S., treatment is approved for patients age eighteen and over for the following:

1. *Myopia—up to -12 diopters. Must be twenty-one or older if greater than 6 diopters.*

2. *Astigmatism—up to 4 diopters as part of a combined myopia and astigmatism procedure (myopic astigmatism). Must be twenty-one or older for more than 1 diopter of astigmatism correction.*

3. *Hyperopia—up to +6 diopters.*

4. *Astigmatism, as part of a combined hyperopia and astigmatism procedure (hyperopic astigmatism) awaits FDA approval.*

Although hyperopic patients, who have up to one diopter of astigmatism in their prescription, are eligible to be treated, the actual laser treatment provides no correction for the astigmatism. Instead, the hyperopia is treated alone. For small amounts of astigmatism this is acceptable. FDA approval for the actual treatment of astigmatism with hyperopia (hyperopic astigmatism) is anticipated before January 1, 2000.

No treatment is available for Presbyopia.

There are other factors that determine whether or not you're a candidate. We'll discuss them in the next chapter.

2
Evaluation of the Potential Excimer Laser Patient

*B*efore we begin our journey into the laser room, we need to know if you're a good candidate. We have just reviewed the biggest factor—determining the type and severity of your refractive error. There are, however, other issues that need to be explored. A comprehensive examination is performed in the office and the items that are discussed and measured include:

A. Your Ocular and Medical History

- What are your visual needs?

- Can you read without glasses?

- How would you feel about wearing reading glasses after the laser treatment?

- Do you have any eye diseases or any medical problems that could affect the outcome?

- **Contraindications,** or conditions, for which the surgery should be avoided:

  1. **Keratoconus** – a very abnormally shaped cornea (figure 14).

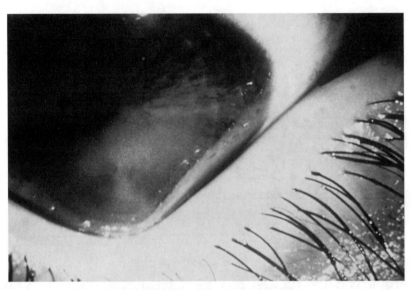

Figure 14— Keratoconus

  2. **Pregnancy or lactation** – high levels of female hormones affect the healing response and can lead to excessive haze and unpredictable results.

  3. **Herpes eye infections.**

  4. **Progressive myopia**
     If the power of your corrective lenses – glasses or contacts – is increasing each year, you have progressive myopia. The laser will permanently correct the present amount but should your eye continue to grow longer you will become more nearsighted.

5. **Active collagen vascular, autoimmune or immunodeficiency diseases,** such as Lupus, Rheumatoid arthritis, or AIDS.

6. **Use of Medications** that can cause corneal scarring or infiltrates, such as Accutane (isoretinoin) and Cordarone (amiodarone).

7. **Presence of cataracts**

There are some conditions that may affect the results of the laser treatment:

a. corneal scars from previous injury or eye surgery, including radial keratotomy.

b. the use of Imitrex (sumatriptin).

c. the formation of prominent large scars from cuts and surgical incisions (patients who are "keloid formers"). This is a problem with PRK, but not with LASIK.

d. diabetes, can cause abnormal healing with general surgical wounds. However, many diabetics have had laser vision surgery with results similar to non-diabetics.

B. Eye Examination

Note: *Before undergoing your eye examination, you must not wear your soft contact lenses for two weeks and your hard or semi-soft, gas-permeable lenses for three weeks. Contact lenses alter the surface of the cornea and can result in faulty measurements of refractive error. While FDA approval required two-week removal of soft contact lenses, many laser surgeons find* *that we get stable measurements on soft lens patients after one week and sometimes after as little as three days. Gas-permeable and hard contact lens wearers, in contrast, can take more than three weeks to stabilize their examination findings.*

The cornea does change its shape in response to a hard contact lens. Some optometrists have tried to reduce a patient's myopia by deliberately fitting contact lenses too tightly to flatten the cornea. This is known as "**orthokeratology**." It does not provide a permanent correction and is limited in creating only small diopter changes.

The eye examination should be thorough and include dilation of the eyes. Included in the testing is the following:

1. Vision Without Glasses or "Uncorrected Visual Acuity"

How well does the person see without his or her glasses or contacts? One eye is measured at a time by covering the other eye with an occluder.

This raises a question that is often asked. What does "**twenty-twenty**" (**20/20**) vision mean? Vision in the U.S. is recorded on a chart with standardized letters, calibrated to be read at a 20-foot distance. We call this measurement your "**visual acuity**." The fraction that describes your vision, i.e. 20/20, 20/40, compares the smallest letters that a person with perfect vision can see at 20 feet to your vision at 20 feet. Therefore, if the ideal subject can see letters at 20 feet, that you can also, your vision is 20/20 (figure 15). However, if you are only capable of seeing larger letters on the chart that can be seen by the "perfect" person standing back 40 feet from it, then your vision is 20/40 (figure 16). Twenty-four hundred vision, 20/400, means

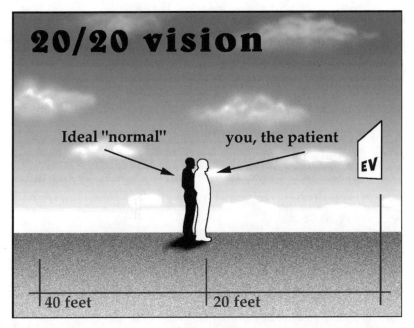

Figure 15

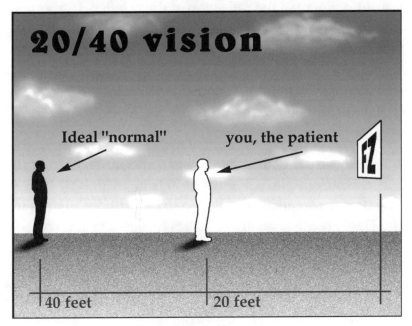

Figure 16

that twenty feet from the chart you can only distinguish the giant E on top, that could be seen by a normal person from 400 feet away. Thus, the bigger the number in the denominator of the fraction describing your visual acuity, (20/60 versus 20/20 for example) the worse your vision.

It is possible to have better than 20/20 vision, although it's unusual. Twenty-fifteen (20/15) vision, means that you can see at 20 feet, letters that a "normally-sighted" person would have to stand 5 feet closer to the chart, or 15 feet away to see.

For those of you who noticed, the exam rooms in the eye doctor's office are not 20 feet long. So how can he record your vision at that distance? The next time you are in the office pay attention to the mirrors on the wall. The letters are projected onto one mirror on the wall behind you, and you read the reflection of those letters in another mirror, 10 feet away on the opposite wall. Pretty tricky. When you have a guest in the exam room with you and the doctor, don't be fooled when that person can read much smaller letters than you can. He is looking directly in the mirror behind you and only seeing the letters from a 10 foot distance.

Some visual acuity levels bear special legal significance. For example, you must be able to see the 20/40 line of letters, or smaller, in order to drive without glasses in the U.S.. For this reason, statistics for laser vision correction are often quoted in relation to the percent of patients achieving 20/40 vision or better. If the best that someone can see with glasses is 20/200 in both eyes, due to a serious eye disease, that person is legally blind.

In the metric system, visual acuity is recorded at 6 meters. Thus 20/20 is written as 6/6, or simply 1, and 20/40 is 0.5.

2. Best Corrected Visual Acuity

What is the best acuity that a person can achieve with glasses or contact lenses? Acuity is measured one eye at a time, covering the other eye with an occluder. We want to make sure that you see normally with glasses. If not, it alerts us to a possible problem with your eyes. Before we jump to any negative conclusions, we perform a refraction to determine if your eyeglass prescription is as good as it can be. This is done two times for patients preparing for laser surgery. The first is referred to as a **manifest refraction**. Dreaded by most patients, this is the most frustrating part of the eye exam for many, choosing between two choices that are similar. "Which is clearer, one or two?" (See figure 17.)

The second measurement for glasses is done after dilating or cycloplegic drops have been instilled in the eyes and given about thirty minutes to work. (See cycloplegic agents pg 5.) This is referred to as a **cycloplegic refraction**. It should confirm the accuracy of the manifest refraction and be almost the same. However, it will reveal whether you were accommodating to focus during the manifest refraction. If you were, you can be prescribed too strong a prescription for glasses, a problem known as "**over-minusing**." We want to set the laser for the minimum myopic correction you need to see 20/20. Otherwise, you can be over-corrected (see pg 61) requiring you to accommodate continually in order to see clearly in the distance, instead of relaxing accommodation and your eye.

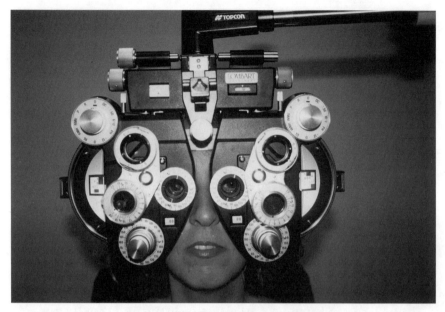

Figure 17—Testing for glasses

An important test for candidacy for the laser treatment is the stability of your refractive error. The refractions described above should be within 0.50 diopters of your old prescription from the previous year. Copies of old contact lens prescriptions or records from previous eye examinations may need to be obtained.

3. Slit Lamp Examination

Your eyes will be examined with an instrument known as a slit lamp microscope that allows a binocular, high magnification view of your eye (figure 18). The cornea is examined to exclude any pathology including keratoconus, scarring, abnormal blood vessels from previous contact lens wear and dry eyes. The crystalline lens is studied to rule out any cloudiness or cataract. Intraocular pressure is measured to screen for glaucoma.

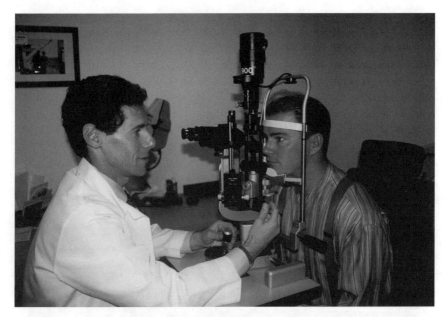

Figure 18-Slit Lamp Microscope exam

4. Keratometry

Your astigmatism may be measured with a keratometer. This measures the power of the flat and steep axis of your cornea. It is very precise, but only uses the central 3 millimeters of your cornea to make its measurements. Newer instrumentation allows a more complete look at the corneal surface (See corneal topography page 28).

5. Retinal Examination

The back of the eye or "retina" is examined to exclude any tears, detachment or predisposing conditions. Patients with high myopia (greater than 6 diopters) are more likely than low myopes or hyperopes to develop retinal pathology. This risk is independent of laser vision correction. The great length of a highly myopic eye can stretch the retina much like canvas being pulled over a frame, and increase the risk of it tearing. The optic nerve that carries vision from the retina to the brain is observed for signs of glaucoma.

6. Corneal Topography or Videokeratography

Astigmatism is nicely demonstrated with this instrument (see figures 6 and 9) as are abnormalities such as keratoconus, where the cornea has an abnormal shape (figure 19).

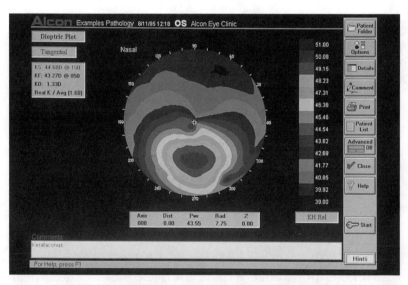

Figure 19—Corneal Topography of Keratoconus
Courtesy of Alcon Surgical

7. Corneal Pachymetry

An ultrasound probe is touched to the surface of the cornea after an eye drop is administered for anesthesia. The thickness of the center of the cornea is measured. This determines the amount of correction that can be obtained. Since the laser ablates or removes some of the corneal tissue and stronger corrections require deeper ablations, we need to know that enough tissue will remain after the treatment for a stable, healthy cornea. Experience over the last seven years has taught us that this residual amount needs to be about 250 microns.

8. Dominant Eye

You may be asked to pretend to aim a gun, or hold a piece of paper with a small hole in it close to your eye to see which one you instinctively depend on as your dominant eye. Some people know without even trying. If one eye is going to be treated at a time instead of having bilateral surgery, the non-dominant eye is often selected for the first treatment.

9. Demonstration of Monovision

If you need reading glasses or are in your late thirties or older, you may be a candidate for "monovision." This refers to using one eye to read and one eye to see in the distance. If you are a myope your non-dominant eye could be left untreated or only given a partial correction to allow you to read without glasses. This option should be discussed and a contact lens used to simulate monovision if you are interested.

10. Informed Consent

One of the most important parts of the comprehensive exam is the informed consent. It is more than a permission slip that you sign for the surgery. The informed consent includes the entire process of educating you about laser vision correction, its risks and benefits. The information provided answers questions such as: what are the chances that you'll be able to see well enough to drive without glasses? What problems could occur during or after the surgery?

If you do not understand something, be sure to ask. We want you to be an informed patient so that you can make the choices that are best for you.

11. Pupil Size

The pupil appears as a black hole, a round opening in your iris — the colored part of the eye. It changes size to adjust the amount of light coming into the eye. In dim light or darkness, it enlarges to allow more light to enter. The size of the pupil, particularily in dim light, will be measured as part of your pre-operative evaluation.

The importance of pupil size relates to a possible side effect of the laser treatment, glare and haloes around lights at night (see pages 65-67). The laser treatment for myopia treats the center of the cornea. If your pupil dilates at night beyond the treated area, you are more likely to experience reduced vision or glare and haloes. Some people have large pupils even in daylight and this needs to be measured as well. The laser treatment for astigmatism with myopia is oval shaped, centered around the pupil. Since the oval is narrower in one direction than the other, it is more likely than myopic treatments without astigmatism to create glare and haloes at night.

3
The Laser Vision Correction Procedures— PRK and LASIK

We've spent some time explaining how we determine whether or not you're a good candidate for laser vision correction. Now we need to describe the two procedures that are performed to help you decide which is best for you. We first need to review some basic anatomy of the cornea.

Anatomy of the Cornea

The cornea is an amazing part of our body; it's a clear window to the eye, similar to the crystal in a watch. How can any human tissue be transparent? The answer lies ahead.

The size of the cornea is 11.5 millimeters in horizontal diameter. Since 25.4 millimeters equals an inch, it is roughly half an inch wide. In its center, the cornea is about 500 microns thick or one half of one millimeter (0.5 mm). That's thin. For comparison, a human hair is about 125 microns thick, so a cornea is roughly the thickness of four hairs.

Under a microscope several layers of the cornea are visible (figure 20). The outermost layer is the **corneal epithelium**, which provides a smooth optical surface that is moistened by tears and functions as a barrier to the germs of the outside world. The thickness of the epithelial layer is about 30 to 50 microns of the total 500. When someone's eye is "scratched" accidently (called a **corneal abrasion**) the epithelium is partially removed (figure 21). Because the corneal nerves run in the epithelium, abrasions are painful. The eye waters and feels like something is lodged in it. Small scratches can heal in a few hours; large ones can take a few days. During the healing process, vision can be very blurry. Comfort is significantly improved by patching the eye closed, covering it with a soft contact "bandage" lens or using topical non-steroidal anti-inflammatory eyedrops (NSAID), such as Acular^{TM} and Voltaren^{TM}. Chemical burns of the eye — acid or alkali — have a similar effect of removing the epithelium, only through chemical rather than mechanical means.

The majority of the cornea is comprised of layers of collagen known as the corneal stroma. Collagen fibers stretch across the cornea and are organized in 200 – 250 layers or lamellae, similar to sheets of paper arranged perpendicularly. The arrangement of the collagen permits light to be transmitted with minimal dispersion by the tissue, allowing the cornea to be transparent.

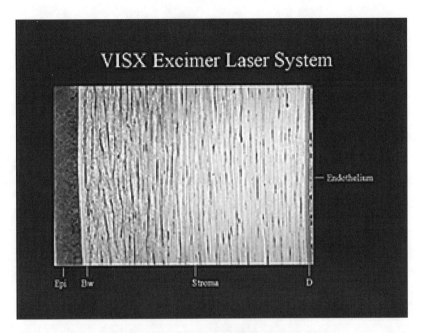

Figure 20—Layers of the cornea
Courtesy of VISX, Inc.

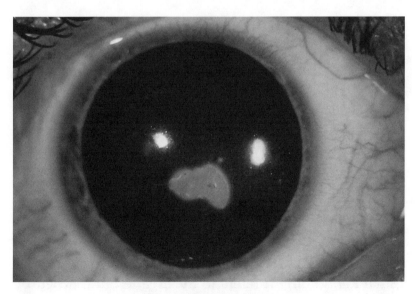

Figure 21—Corneal abrasion

The innermost structure of the cornea is the **endothelial cell layer**. These cells pump water out of the cornea and keep it from swelling with fluid from the inside of the eye. Endothelial cells are critical to the health of the cornea. For an eye surgery to be safe, these cells need to be preserved. Some people have a condition known as corneal guttata where they have fewer endothelial cells than are normal. **Fuch's Corneal Dystrophy** is a hereditary condition with a progressive loss of endothelial cells.

Radial Keratotomy (RK)

Before discussing laser corneal refractive procedures, an earlier operation deserves mention. Radial keratotomy is of importance not only from a historical perspective, but also because many incorrectly assume it to be related to PRK and LASIK.

Radial keratotomy, or **"RK,"** uses radial incisions to flatten the cornea to correct myopia (figure 22). It is also known as **"incisional refractive surgery."** A hand-held diamond knife is used to perform the operation. The central cornea, over the pupil, is marked with a circular ring. Corneal thickness is measured in the operating room with an ultrasound pachymeter and a diamond blade is extended to the appropriate length. Incisions are made from the optical zone mark out to the periphery of the cornea, sparing the center.

This introduces a common term that pertains to all corneal refractive surgeries, the **optical zone** size. For radial keratotomy it refers to the area left untouched by any incisions. For laser vision correction it refers to the size of the area of the central cornea treated by the surgery, measuring outward from the center of the pupil. When a three millimeter ring is centered over the pupil then pressed lightly on the cornea, it leaves a circle three millimeters in diameter. The area outlined by this mark is referred to as the three millimeter optical zone. Similarly, four, five, six and seven millimeter rings mark corresponding optical zone sizes.

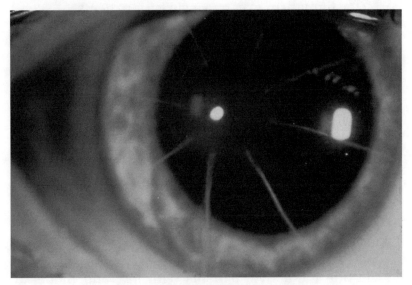

Figure 22—Radial Keratotomy

There are three variables that control the amount of correction obtained with RK. The first is the size of the optical zone. Incisions made closer to the center of the cornea have more effect. The second variable is the number of incisions — four, eight and unadvisably sixteen. More incisions give more correction. The third is the depth of the incisions. Deep cuts are required to get a good effect.

Charts are constructed of the average diopters of correction obtained for the various optical zone sizes and number of incisions. These tables are referred to as "**nomograms**." Each surgeon would start with an experienced surgeon's nomogram and fine tune his own, based on personal surgical results.

Astigmatism can be corrected with a diamond knife by making a pair of incisions in the steep axis. This is called "**astigmatic keratotomy**" **or** "**AK**" and is also used to correct astigmatism in cataract surgery patients.

Radial keratotomy is limited in its accuracy by the individual healing response of the patient. In some the incisions have healed more tightly than expected based on the information from the nomograms, resulting in less effect. Others have not healed as well as expected and were over-treated causing hyperopia. In many cases the correction obtained continued to increase over the years, a process known as "**hyperopic shift**." Fluctuation in vision could occur between day and night because the pressure in the eye changes and pushes out on the incisions in varying degrees.

Despite the above, patients with low and moderate myopia are quite pleased with their RK results. Patients with myopia higher than seven diopters have never done as well. Attempts to correct these patients with a large number of incisions, sometimes sixteen or more, weakened the cornea and led to unpredictable outcomes.

Radial keratotomy was, and still is, a viable procedure for the correction of low degrees of myopia and astigmatism. Laser vision correction, in my opinion, is a better choice. Since the availability of the excimer laser, I have not performed RK on any of my patients.

Photorefractive Keratectomy (PRK)

The history books will state, "and then came the laser." The precision of this computerized instrument for performing corneal surgery is unsurpassed. To appreciate this, look at the photograph of a pattern carved by the laser on a human hair (figure 23).

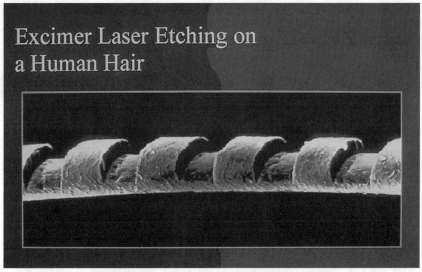

Excimer Laser Etching on a Human Hair

Figure 23—Courtesy of VISX and IBM

The excimer laser uses invisible ultra-violet light. This cool light produces negligible thermal damage to the surrounding tissue. Each pulse of the laser removes only 0.25 microns of corneal tissue, or 1/500th of the thickness of a human hair per pulse (figure 24). Remember that though the center of the cornea varies, it is about 500 microns thick, and a hair is about 125 microns. Thus, it would take 500 pulses to cut through a human hair and 2,000 to penetrate the cornea. The laser removes tissue by the breakdown of molecular bonds, a process known as **photoablation**.

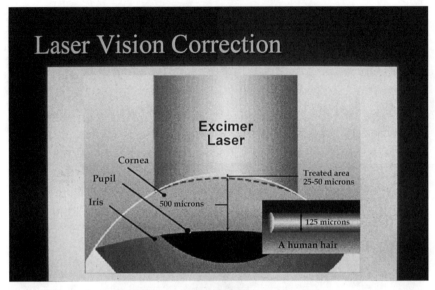

Figure 24

A Description of the PRK Procedure

To correct myopia the cornea needs to be weakened by flattening its surface. This is accomplished by excising or ablating the central corneal tissue. The more correction required, the deeper the ablation that is performed. To access the stroma, the covering epithelium needs to be removed. Let's walk through a case:

The laser is generally located in an office or surgery center. When you arrive for your surgery you will be greeted by an assistant who will explain the procedure to you and answer any questions. If only one eye is being treated, as is typical for PRK, an adhesive paper marker such as a gold star will be placed on your forehead above your operative eye. You will be given a pill to relax you, typically valium. Antibiotic, anesthetic and anti-inflammatory drops are then instilled in the operative eye.

If you have astigmatism, you may be taken into a separate room to have the horizontal or vertical axis of your eye marked. A fine tip felt pen is used to make two or more dots horizontally and/or vertically on the white of your eye, next to the cornea. This allows us to make sure your eye is properly oriented and not rotated when you lie down under the laser.

You will then be escorted into the laser room, a room carefully controlled for temperature and humidity. One of the interesting things we have learned over the last seven years is that the environment, including altitude, affects the correction the laser can achieve. When the humidity is high, less correction is obtained. Lasers in Denver, the "mile-high city," use less energy (fewer pulses) to achieve the same ablation as lasers at sea level. The laser has delicate optics (lenses and mirrors) that are sensitive to organic compounds, including perfume. You will be asked not to wear any cologne the day of your surgery. Regular hospital cleaning crews are generally forbidden from entering the laser room because of the harsh organic cleaning compounds they use.

The surgeon and several technicians and assistants will be in the laser room. One will help guide you onto the laser bed (figure 25) and will position your head correctly. Another will be responsible for calibrating the laser output and verifying its accuracy. The same person will enter the prescription to be corrected into the computer and will verify it with the surgeon. A third technician will assist the doctor by passing the instruments to him from a sterile tray.

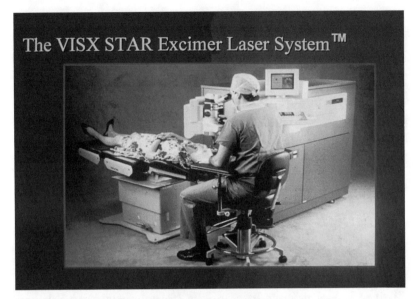

**Figure 25—Patient and surgeon in position
Courtesy of VISX, Inc.**

The laser has a microscope with adjustable brightness to allow the surgeon to see your eye clearly under high magnification. Each laser manufacturer has its own system to ensure that the eye is centered under the laser. They all involve maintaining your pupil in the center of a reticule or between two aligning beams (figure 26). If astigmatism is being treated, the marks made on the white of your eye can be aligned with the horizontal marks of the reticule.

The laser technician will call your attention to a popping, metallic sound. When the laser fires it creates an acoustic shock wave that causes this noise. It does not hurt however. Before your procedure begins, the technician will fire a few test shots to check the power output or **fluence** of the laser.

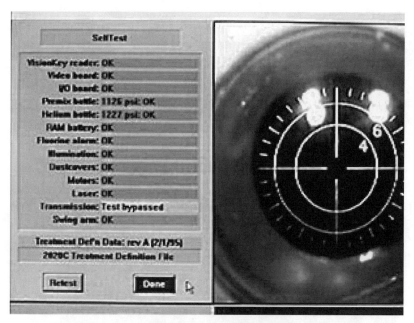

**Figure 26—Reticule to monitor patient fixation
Courtesy of VISX, Inc.**

A wire speculum is used to spread apart the upper and lower eyelids in order to hold your eye open during the procedure (figure 27). Another anesthetic drop is instilled in your eye and your other eye is patched closed. You will then be asked to look at the red light, the infra-red aiming beam of the laser. The laser light itself is not visible in most lasers.

The surgeon will center a circular marker with a 7 millimeter diameter around your pupil. He will use this to make a light indentation in the corneal epithelium. This will create a 7 millimeter optical zone marking (see page 34). An instrument is used to wipe off the epithelium outlined by this mark. Great care is taken to remove all of the epithelium. The amount of time spent removing the epithelium is important as well. The longer the surgeon takes to complete this step the more the cornea will dry. The degree of hydration of the cornea affects the outcome. The drier the cornea becomes, the greater is the correction achieved. You do not need to concentrate on the red light during the epithelial removal.

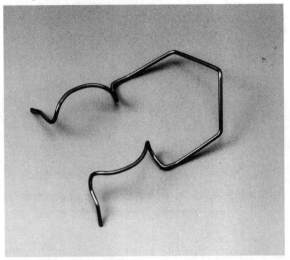

Figure 27—Eyelid Speculum
Courtesy of Bausch & Lomb Surgical

You are now ready for the actual laser procedure. The surgeon will alert you to this fact and ask again for your cooperation in viewing the red light. He then presses down on a foot pedal, similar to a gas pedal in a car, and the treatment begins. You will hear a suction noise and you will be aware of a clicking sound. During the ablation of the corneal tissue a burning odor is given off, and the suction tube helps capture the vapor and smell.

The length of the actual laser treatment varies from 30 to 90 seconds depending on the strength of your prescription, the amount of tissue that needs to be ablated, and the specific laser used. An ablation of approximately 12 microns equates to a correction of 1 diopter and takes 8 seconds or 48 pulses of the laser to complete. The exact depth varies with each laser manufacturer as does the time for treatment, since different lasers operate at different frequencies or pulses delivered per second. Should your eye move off center from the aiming reticule or aligning beams, the surgeon will release his foot from the pedal and stop the laser. Some new lasers now have trackers that follow the eye (see chapter 6). You will be asked to again focus on the light and the laser will resume treatment where it left off.

While the laser is firing, the technician will often count off how much time remains so you have an idea of the progress. Another assistant will hold your hand.

When the laser is complete a bandage contact lens is applied to the eye and antibiotic and steroid drops are again instilled. The lid speculum is removed and you will slowly get up and walk into the recovery area. Congratulations! You're going to see the world through new eyes.

Recovery from PRK

As described above, the central 6 to 7 millimeters of the corneal epithelium is removed for PRK. This creates a situation equivalent to a scratched eye or corneal abrasion that causes irritation and watering of the eye and blurry vision as well. To minimize these symptoms a soft contact lens with no or minimal prescription may be used. As mentioned above, this is known as a **bandage contact lens**. This lens is left in place for about four days, until the epithelium has healed underneath. You will be given special non-steroidal anti-inflammatory drops (NSAID), Ocufen™ or Acular™, which will greatly help with comfort.

You will be asked to come into the office daily or every other day until the contact lens is removed. During this time you will be using the NSAID, steroid and antibiotic drops. The frequency of these drops will be determined by your physician and will be reduced over the next several weeks. Your vision will be blurry the first few days, but once the corneal epithelium has healed and the bandage lens removed, it will be much better. By one week, your vision will be reasonably good. The healing response continues, however, over the next few months. By three months the correction is stable.

An aside about **"steroid drops."** Understandably, many patients are frightened when the hear the word "steroid." Eyedrops use low concentrations of these medications and are very minimally absorbed into the body. They drain down the tear duct into your nose and some absorption occurs there. This is why you may taste the eye drops in the back of your throat. The only potential side effects involve your eye. Long-term use by some patients can cause an elevated eye pressure or glaucoma, and/or cataracts. The pressure elevation goes away when the drops are stopped, but any damage done is permanent.

Wall Street Disappointed by PRK

Although the results of PRK are excellent, it is easy to see why patients have not flocked by the millions to have this procedure performed. Imagine that a friend in your office has had PRK. You're nearsighted and anxious to find out how she did. You call her the night of surgery:

You: "How'd it go?"

Susan: "OK."

You: "Can you see?"

Susan: "Well...It's kind of blurry."

You: "Did it hurt?"

Susan: "Not when they did it, but now it does. It feels like there's something in my eye and it keeps watering."

You: "Oh. (pause) I hope you feel better soon."

Initial projections by Wall Street analysts following FDA approval in October 1995, predicted between 750,000 and one million PRK procedures. This was based on the number of myopes in the U.S. You can understand, based on the initial recovery period, why PRK failed to "meet the street." Approximately, 80,000 PRK procedures were performed in 1996. Stock prices for laser manufacturers plummetted.

LASIK—the Wow Factor!

The situation has changed dramatically in the last two years. Once underutilized, laser centers are now operating full speed. The change is due in part to growing consumer awareness about laser vision correction in general, but the most important factor is the growing popularity of a procedure known as LASIK. This acronym stands for Laser in Situ Keratomileusis. Forget what that means. You'll better understand an expression used by physicians to describe LASIK, which is "**flap and zap**."

LASIK has what PRK was missing—the *WOW* factor—and this is responsible for the dramatic increase in the number of patients undergoing laser vision correction. In 1997 the number of LASIK and PRK procedures combined rose to 200,000. That many cases were performed in the first half of 1998, [1] and estimates are between 350,000 [2] and 500,000 [1] for the entire year. Now imagine *this* phone call between you and your friend:

You: "How'd it go today?"

Susan: "Great!"

You: "Can you see?"

Susan: "Yes. I can't believe it. I'm sitting here watching TV without my glasses."

You: "Did it hurt?"

Susan: "Not really. I felt some pressure but it only lasted a minute."

You: "I'm glad you did so well. What did you say that doctor's name was?"

That's the *WOW* factor at work.

What Makes LASIK so Special?

LASIK uses the same excimer laser as PRK to perform an ablation of the corneal stroma. The difference is that the laser is applied beneath a superficial lamellar flap of corneal tissue (figure 28). The process of creating or cutting a corneal flap is known as a **keratectomy** and the instrument that makes the incision a **microkeratome** (figure 29). The flap is left attached to the cornea by a hinge, which is made by having the microkeratome stop before it fully traverses

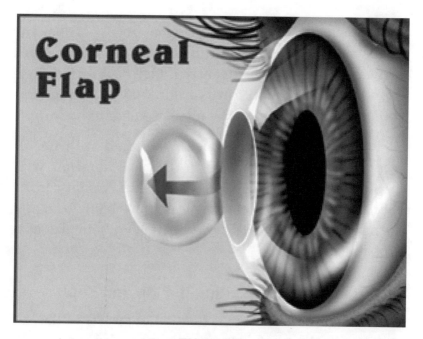

Figure 28

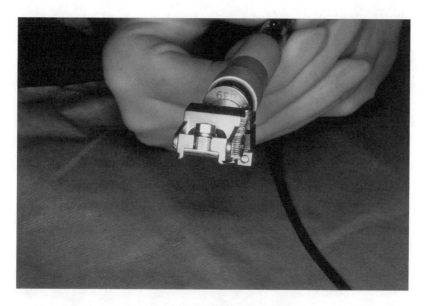

Figure 29—Microkeratome

the diameter of the cornea, leaving an uncut portion. The flap is usually 160 or 180 microns of the 550 micron thick cornea. For the laser treatment, it is bent back on its hinge. Afterwards, it is replaced in its original position. It adheres by itself, without sutures, by force of suction.

Less healing of the surface is required with LASIK compared to PRK. There is no corneal abrasion with LASIK and no bandage lens is needed. Vision can be checked five minutes later; typically it's about 20/70. By the next morning 20/40 vision or better, without glasses is probable.

WOW! Now You're Getting it. Flap and Zap!

With LASIK it has become common to perform **bilateral surgery**, treating both eyes on the same day. Let's walk through a LASIK procedure:

The pre-operative drops and sedation will be the same as described for PRK (see pg 38). You will be positioned on the laser bed as described before. The technician who hands the surgeon the instruments assembles the microkeratome, which has several pieces (figure 30). There are a number of manufacturers of keratomes and different models, but I'll describe one of the more commonly used instruments. Great care is taken when handling the disposable blade (figure 31), to avoid any damage to it's cutting edge, which should be checked under the microscope before use. A depth plate is chosen that determines the thickness of the flap that the blade will cut, usually 160 or 180 microns.

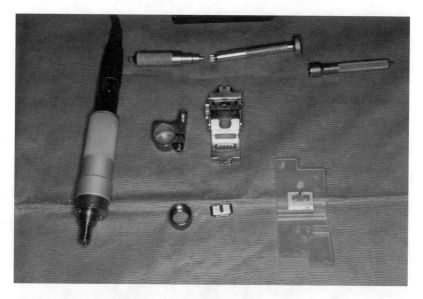

Figure 30—Unassembled microkeratome

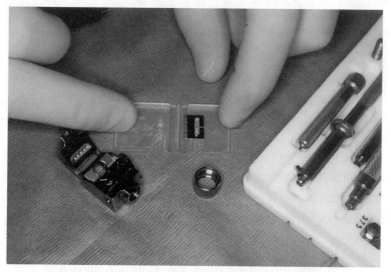

Figure 31—Disposable microkeratome blade

Before it is placed on the eye, the keratome is positioned on the suction ring (figure 32). The foot pedal is activated to verify proper movement across the track. The suction ring is also tested, by occluding its port with a finger to check that the vacuum rises to an appropriate level.

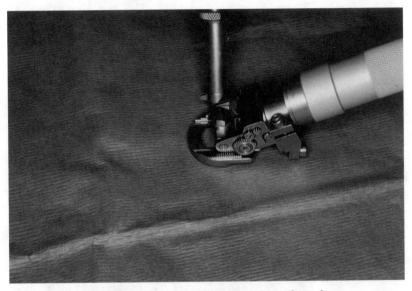

Figure 32—Microkeratome on suction ring.

The laser technician checks the fluence or energy output of the laser. You will hear a clanging noise as the laser fires to calibrate itself . Once the surgeon and the technician have completed their testing the procedure is ready to begin.

Your eyelashes are covered with a plastic drape and a speculum is inserted to hold your eyelids open. Your opposite eye is patched closed. You are asked to focus on the red light and a special marker is centered over your pupil. Gentian violet dye is applied to the undersurface of the marker so that a colored mark is left on the corneal surface. In the event that no hinge is made during the keratectomy and a **"free cap"** is created, see page 75, the mark left on the cornea would allow proper orientation of the cap back on the eye.

The next step is placement of the suction ring on the eye. Similar to a donut, the ring has a large central hole which is centered over the entire cornea. Good exposure of the eye is required for proper placement of the ring. Some patients have prominent eyes that protrude well and lids that open widely. Others have deep set eyes or narrow lid fissures that prevent wide exposure.

Once the surgeon has adequate exposure and good positioning of the suction ring, he calls for the assistant to turn on the suction. The surgeon usually does not control the footpedal so that he does not inadvertently turn off the suction during the keratectomy.

It is normal to feel some pressure when the suction is turned on and for your vision to go dim or black. A special instrument is used to verify that the eye pressure is raised to a sufficient level. An assistant calls out the pressure while the suction is on, to assure the surgeon that it is being maintained.

Next the surgeon places the microkeratome on its track on the suction ring. The track is inspected to exclude and remove anything that could get in the way of the passage of the microkeratome, such as drape material, lid speculum, or eyelid. If anything were to obstruct the passage of the keratome, an incomplete flap would be cut and the procedure aborted. The footpedal is then pressed to start the automated keratome on its way. Once it progresses across the cornea, the stop, a metal pin on the keratome, hits against the suction ring and ceases the foward movement. This prevents the microkeratome from moving completely across the cornea and creating a free cap. Only a few seconds are required for the microkeratome to cut the flap. The suction is turned off, then the ring and keratome are lifted off the eye. The flap is lifted, inspected for quality, and bent back out of the way (figure 33).

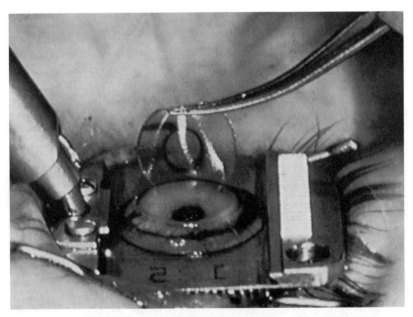

Figure 33—LASIK—lifting the flap
Photo courtesy Richard Lindstrom, M.D.

It is now time for the excimer ablation. This proceeds the same as described for PRK after the epithelium has been removed. The laser ablation lasts thirty to ninety seconds, as with PRK. The flap is then repositioned. Sterile saline on a cannula is used to irrigate in the plane between the flap and the underlying corneal stromal bed. The irrigation has a two-fold purpose. One is to flush out any debris which might otherwise accumulate in the interface. This debris is not visually significant. The other is to allow the cap to orient back exactly as it was before the cut, floating in place on a thin layer of fluid, which runs out as the cornea settles in its original position.

In a matter of minutes the flap adheres. The surface of the cornea is gently stroked with a cellulose sponge to encourage the process. After three to five minutes a final check is made. If the flap is centered, with no folds or "**striae**," the procedure is over. The lid speculum is carefully removed to avoid any contact with the flap. You are asked to blink your eye and the flap is examined once more. Many doctors will examine you in ten to twenty minutes using a slit lamp (see pg 27) in another room of the office or laser center.

If your other eye is to have surgery, the entire process is repeated. The entire procedure as described above, takes about ten minutes per eye. Therefore, bilateral surgery is completed in twenty to twenty-five minutes.

Recovery and Healing of LASIK

LASIK does indeed have the *WOW* factor. It amazes patients and brings them tears of joy. They are unable to believe the immediacy of their results and their new found freedom to see.

The exam on the morning following surgery is the most important. The flap is examined for proper position and absence of folds. If there is any irregularity, it needs to be lifted and repositioned as described above for the initial LASIK procedure.

Since the epithelium is not removed for LASIK, there is no epithelial defect to heal. This means greater comfort for the patient. Antibiotic and steroid drops are used for one to three weeks, depending on the surgeon's preference. This is far less than the three month period for PRK.

Vision the morning after surgery is commonly 20/40 or better without glasses. Patients with astigmatism and high myopes are a little slower to recover vision this sharp. The results for the varying degrees of myopia and astigmatism are reviewed in chapter five.

One of the great things about LASIK as compared to PRK is that problems related to corneal haze are virtually non-existent. That's great news for all patients but especially for the higher myopes who are prone to develop haze.

Retreatment

If **retreatment** is necessary due to an undercorrection or overcorrection, there are two options. One is to dissect and free the edge of the original corneal flap and peel it back open, then apply more laser. The other is to cut an entirely new flap. Preference varies among surgeons and is partly dependent on the amount of time that has elapsed since surgery. The greater the time that has passed, the more likely that a new flap will be cut.

Maximum Limit of Myopia Correction with LASIK

What is the maximum limit of correction obtainable with LASIK? It actually varies from one patient to another, but typically it is somewhere around 12 diopters of myopia.

Experience has taught us that 250 microns must remain in the corneal bed after the excimer ablation to allow a stable corneal shape. If a patient has a 550 micron cornea and the surgeon cuts a 160 micron flap, 390 microns remain in the bed. In order to leave 250 behind, up to 140 microns could be excised. That equals approximately 11.6 diopters of maximum correction. But if the same patient's cornea is 500 microns thick, only 90 microns could be excised or 7.5 diopters corrected.

Nomograms: Dealing with Variations in Results

Surgeons develop their own nomograms for LASIK, as with RK. This involves comparing the achieved results with the intended corrections in order to arrive at an adjustment factor. The full amount of your refractive error is generally not entered into the laser. Nomograms refer to tables listing the adjustment factor — by age and degree of myopia — by which to reduce your prescription for the laser treatment. Small variations in technique among surgeons, such as how dry or moist the cornea is kept and differences in the energy output of individual lasers, as well as the humidity and temperature in the laser room, will alter the outcome of the procedure. With time a surgeon becomes familiar with the results of his laser and creates his own adjustment factor to fine tune the results.

Unilateral Versus Bilateral Surgery

A conservative approach is to operate on one eye at a time or unilaterally. This provides the opportunity to observe the healing response and make adjustments, if needed, to the treatment plan for the second eye. Of course, the amount of time that passes between the two surgeries is a factor. One week gives some clue to the final correction obtained but is still premature. After three to four weeks, the final result is more secure for LASIK. Few patients are willing to wait that long, and if the surgery is done one eye at a time, the second eye is usually treated one week after the first.

A contact lens can be worn in the unoperated eye or one lens can be popped out of the eyeglasses. For some patients this is intolerable and may interfere with their jobs. For convenience, many patients choose bilateral sequential surgery. First one eye is treated, then the other, minutes apart. The excellence of the LASIK procedure in skilled hands makes this a viable option.

FDA Approval

Until recently the U.S. was a few years behind the rest of the world in PRK and LASIK because of the Food and Drug Administration (FDA). FDA research is a mixed blessing to medical science. On the one hand it is a conservative mechanism providing for the careful study of new procedures. This is important for public safety. On the other hand , the process slows progress tremendously, sometimes jeopardizing the very public it seeks to protect. Also the costs involved for companies trying to develop new products is prohibitive. Many times a company will decide not to proceed with further development of a product. When a company does go ahead with years of testing, guess who pays? You! The ultimate cost of the new drug or procedure will reflect the development costs.

Approval for excimer laser PRK did not come until 1995. It should be comforting for you to know how much time and effort went into assuring its safety.

LASIK has developed from PRK, adding the keratectomy step. FDA approval is being sought. In the meantime it is allowed as an "off label" use of the excimer laser. Permission forms for surgery or the "informed consent" must reflect discussion of the "off label" use of the laser.

References

1. Moretti, M., and Harmon, D., "Laser Vision Correction Volume Continues Strong Growth," *EyeWorld*, volume 3, number 12, pgs. 14 and 24, December 1998.

2. "Refractive Surgery Surges," in *Review of Ophthalmology*, September 1998, pg. 4.

4
Is it Safe?

*O*ne of the most important questions concerns the safety of laser vision correction. Just as the FDA had to be assured, so do you. The answer to the safety question, in my opinion, is "yes" for PRK, and "Yes, in experienced hands or under qualified supervision," for LASIK.

The word "safe" is problematic. Everyday usage is different from the way trial attorneys take advantage of it in court. Does "safe" mean that absolutely nothing can go wrong? In my opinion, no. We routinely travel on airplanes and in cars. Is it safe? In the opinion of this author, yes. All of us are aware that serious accidents do occur; we could even die in a crash. But the relative odds are way in our favor. More common are problems of delayed flights or equipment malfunction requiring change in aircraft. The same is true for laser vision correction. In a rare situation there could be serious loss of vision. However, most of the time nothing goes wrong and when it does, it is manageable. The discussion that follows will review this.

Statistics shown on PRK complications are from VISX, Inc.[1] VISX gathered data on a large group of PRK patients followed for at least two years, and presented it to the FDA for approval. Published statistics on LASIK are generally on fewer patients followed for a shorter length of time.

This chapter is not intended as (nor does it claim to be) a formalized review of all studies published in the medical literature. Its purpose is to present an overview of the safety of the procedures.

What are the possible complications of laser vision correction?

When the cornea is ablated by the laser, a healing response is stimulated. As discussed with radial keratotomy (see pg 36), variations in the healing of the cornea can affect the amount of correction obtained, and thus the accuracy of the surgery. With PRK, the results in large numbers of patients have been outstanding. (This will be reviewed in chapter 5.) In any individual patient, however, healing is a variable.

Complications Due to the *Laser* Component of the Procedure:

1. Undercorrection

The laser correction might not be as much as intended. After stabilization, additional laser may need to be applied. As discussed earlier, many factors affect the result: the healing response of the eye, the hydration of the cornea during the procedure, the individual laser and its calibration, and the temperature and humidity of the laser room. If needed, additional laser treatment, or **retreatment**, can be added after three months when the results of PRK have stabilized.

If the undercorrection is deliberate in order to create "**monovision**" — leaving the patient with residual myopia in one eye to allow reading vision — it would not be considered a complication.

With a single PRK treatment, 83.6 percent (363 of 434 eyes) of myopes up to 6 diopters were within 1 diopter of the intended correction at one month following the procedure. By six months the percent within this range had risen to 91.6 (384 of 419 eyes).[1] After six months the results were stable.

For LASIK in the same range of myopia (up to 6 diopters) 95 percent of patients were within 1 diopter at one month and one year.[2] LASIK data for this study was on 236 patients with low myopia, 191 of which were studied at one month, and only 44 of which had made it to the one year mark at the time the data were reported.

Retreatment, for enhancement — to add more correction — was performed in 2.1 percent of the low myopia group of LASIK patients.[2]

The accuracy of the laser treatments can better be appreciated by studying the visual results (see chapter 5).

2. Overcorrection

The laser correction may exceed the desirable level, converting a myope into a hyperope. This used to be a more serious problem than undercorrection, since no effective treatment was readily available to correct hyperopia. This has changed, however, with the approval of PRK for hyperopia.

At two years, 1.3 percent of PRK treated eyes (7 out of 542) were overtreated by more than 1 diopter and 0.6 percent (3 out of 542) by more than 2 diopters.[1] Results were similar one year after surgery.

3. Induced or Incompletely Treated Astigmatism

The correction of astigmatism has always been more difficult than the treatment of myopia. Rather than uniformly modifying the surface of the cornea, one specific axis must be changed more than the rest. Astigmatism has previously been described as a corneal surface that is not round. There are, however, some patients who have a round or spherical cornea, but whose crystalline lens is astigmatic (lenticular astigmatism). The laser can correct either type of astigmatism, but can only do so by making changes in the cornea, since the lens is not treated.

If the axis of astigmatism being corrected is off – 100 degrees instead of 90 for example – then a new astigmatism will occur in a different axis or direction. When you lie down on the laser table your eye can tort or rotate, so what appears to the surgeon to be vertical is not. Your eye needs to be aligned in the laser to make sure that straight up and down on the laser reticule is aligned with up and down on your eye. Some surgeons use an absorbable felt tip pen to mark the horizontal or vertical axis of your eye to help in orientation. Other surgeons use some landmark on the eye to guide them, such as a blood vessel or a freckle.

Another problem that can occur is creation of astigmatism in an eye that had none prior to treatment. The cause is not well understood. A combination of factors might contribute such as the alignment of the patient's eye and the evenness or "**homogeneity** "of the laser beam. This same problem occured with radial keratotomy as well, where no laser beam was used. Fortunately, the amount of astigmatism created is generally small with little effect on uncorrected visual acuity. At twelve and twenty four months after PRK for up to 6 diopters, 3.0 percent of eyes (16 eyes out of 542) had an increase of 1 or more diopters in their astigmatism, but none increased by 2 or more diopters.[1]

A more serious problem is creation of irregular astigmatism (see pg. 10). If the surface is left with any unevenness after PRK, you can have irregular astigmatism. In LASIK the keratectomy can create irregular astigmatism if the flap does not lie down smoothly in its exact original position. Irregular astigmatism will reduce your visual acuity and you may be required to wear gas permeable contact lenses to achieve the best possible vision.

For all of the above reasons, the correction of astigmatism with the laser, while quite accurate, may not be as excellent as the correction of the myopia component. Since most patients have much more myopia than they do astigmatism, the net result of laser vision correction is excellent.

4. Corneal Haze

The normal response of the cornea to PRK is to heal. If that response is exaggerated, the cornea can develop **haze**, or a ground glass appearance (figure 34). Haze is visible under high magnification, not to the naked eye. It can be reduced or eliminated by the use of topical corticosteroid eyedrops. Corneal haze is almost never seen with LASIK, which explains why LASIK patients are taken off their drops much sooner than those treated by PRK.

In most instances haze is mild and not visually significant. More dense haze can blur your vision and result in loss of correction or "regression." This means that your myopia will return to some degree. It may be enough to require retreatment with the laser to eliminate the haze and return the proper correction. Because healing of PRK takes several months to stabilize, retreatment is not recommended for at least three months. During this time, patients are usually maintained on steroid eyedrops.

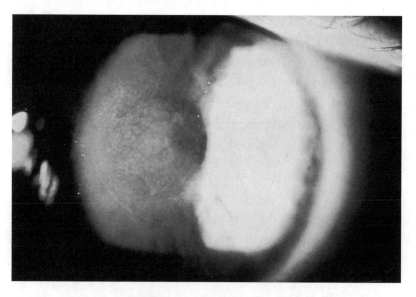

Figure 34—Corneal haze
Photo courtesy Richard Lindstrom, M.D.

A total of 3.6 percent of eyes were re-treated over the course of the VISX FDA study of low to moderate myopes[1] For high myopia of 6 to 12 diopters, 1.5 percent (3 of 200 eyes) were retreated for regression, haze and irregular astigmatism.[1]

The amount of myopia being corrected is associated with both the risk of developing haze and its severity. Since haze occurs as an exaggeration of the healing response, more myopia, requiring deeper surgery, equals higher risk and greater haze. This has led to the suggestion by some surgeons that PRK be reserved for lower to moderate myopes and LASIK be used for higher. Most surgeons are using LASIK for all of their patients regardless of their degree of myopia.

Haze is graded as:

- 0.0 to 0.5 = trace

- 1.0 to 1.5 = mild

- 2.0 = moderate

- 3.0 = severe

Statistics show that at one year, for patients up to 6 diopters of myopia treated by PRK, 0.6 percent (3 of 520 eyes) had grade 2 or higher haze.[1] This reduced to 0.2 percent (1 of 542 eyes) by two years. For high myopia of 6 to 12 diopters treated by PRK, 1.3 percent had corneal haze with loss of two or more lines of best corrected vision at a twelve month follow up. In a study of astigmatism patients treated by PRK 1.2 percent (1 of 82 eyes) had grade 2 or higher haze at two years.

5. Decreased Night Vision/ Haloes and Starbursts

We do not see as well at night as we do during the day. Our retina has two types of receptors, cones and rods. Cones are responsible for our sharpest vision and color perception. In darkness, rods provide us with most of our vision.

Both PRK and LASIK are associated with reduced vision at night, mostly experienced as glare and starbursts around lights. Some patients describe this as similar to their nightime vision with contact lenses, but many have no complaints.

Significant lessening of the occurence and severity of these problems has been accomplished by increasing the size of the optical zone. If you recall, the optical zone is the size of a circular area centered around the pupil that is treated by the laser. Our pupils dilate at night, and our eyes have to focus light coming in more peripherally or farther from the center of the cornea. The larger the optical zone of laser treatment, the greater the corneal surface area that will be available to focus light in these conditions.

Early on, PRK treatments were done with smaller optical zone sizes, below 6 millimeters. Once the technology improved to allow larger optical zone treatment, the incidence of troublesome glare and starbursts decreased. Data supplied to the FDA show that between 4 to 5 percent of patients with low to moderate myopia (up to 6 diopters) have more difficulty with night vision after treatment than before, when questioned from three months to two years after surgery.[1] Sensitivity to bright lights was reported in 3.0 percent (16 of 542 eyes) and "double vision" in 1.3 percent (7 of 542 eyes) after two years. Night time glare and starbursts can be a problem after laser vision correction.

In a much smaller group of 116 patients treated for astigmatism by PRK, the results were worse. At two years, 22.6 percent (19 of 82 eyes) reported more trouble with night vision after the surgery than before, and 15.5 percent (13 of 82) reported greater sensitivity to bright lights.

6. Decentered Ablation

If the laser treatment is not centered around the pupil, the results will be less than desired. Some of the light entering the eye will be focused properly and some will not. This can reduce vision.

You need to fixate on the aiming beam of the laser, and the physician needs to monitor that this is being done properly. If your head is not perpendicular to the laser beam, it may appear that the laser is centered when in actuality it is not. Patients have a tendency to drop their chins toward their chests as the procedure progresses. The surgeon is always alert for this. If you lose focus, or your head is not properly aligned, the treatment will be temporarily stopped and the situation corrected, then the treatment will be resumed.

7. Infection

Although rare, infection can cause a corneal ulcer after PRK (figure 35). This can result in scarring, which might reduce your best corrected acuity. Preventative measures are taken such as using antibiotic eye drops. This is particularly important the first week following PRK, while waiting for the corneal epithelium to heal. The epithelium is the barrier that prevents germs from getting to deeper layers of the cornea. A corneal ulcer can lead to scarring and, in the most extreme situations, a surface irregular enough to require a corneal transplant.

In the FDA study of VISX laser patients treated for low to moderate myopia, three patients suffered a corneal ulcer or infiltrate within a month after surgery. No infections occured after this and there was no loss of vision. Because the corneal epithelium is only minimally disrupted with LASIK, the chance of a corneal infection is much less.

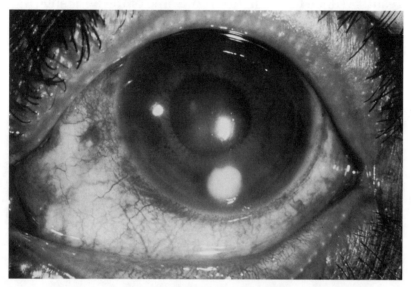

Figure 35—Corneal ulcer

8. Loss of Best Corrected Visual Acuity

Uncorrected and best corrected visual acuity were discussed previously on pages 22-26. The purpose of laser vision correction is to improve your uncorrected distance visual acuity. It is presumed that following laser surgery you could wear glasses or contact lenses and achieve the best vision that you had pre-operatively. For example, say your vision is 20/400 without glasses and 20/20 with them. After laser surgery, your uncorrected visual acuity may improve to 20/30. Nearly perfect. It is expected that with a new prescription for thinner eyeglasses you could still enjoy 20/20 vision.

Loss of best spectacle corrected visual acuity (loss of BSCVA) is a complication of great concern which has been studied intently by the FDA. If you undergo laser surgery and see 20/30 without glasses, but cannot be made to see any better with new glasses, then you have lost best corrected acuity. You were 20/20 best corrected with glasses before the surgery, but only 20/30 after. This is disappointing despite the improvement of your uncorrected visual acuity from 20/400 to 20/30.

In discussing this topic and gathering statistics, we refer to the number of lines of acuity which were lost. The lines on the eye chart start with the smallest letters at the bottom, the 20/15 line. They increase in size to 20/20, then 20/25, 20/30, 20/40, 20/50, 20/60, 20/70, 20/80, 20/100, 20/200 and 20/400.

Thus, if you drop from a best corrected acuity of 20/20 pre-operatively to 20/30 post-operatively, you have lost two lines of vision. In other words the best you can see with glasses is two lines higher on the chart after surgery than before. In studying this complication, significant loss of vision is usually considered to be loss of two or more lines.

Many factors, as discussed above, can result in a loss of best corrected visual acuity. The creation of irregular astigmatism, corneal haze, infection, scarring, and any problems related to the corneal flap can all contribute. Many of these will improve with time.

For myopia up to 6 diopters treated by PRK, after twenty-four months only 0.2 percent (1 of 542) of treated eyes had loss of two lines or more best spectacle corrected visual acuity.[1] After 12 months for high myopia of 6 to 12 diopters treated by PRK, 5.8 percent (9 of 156) of eyes lost two or more lines of BSCVA.[1]

In comparison, in one study of LASIK for myopia up to 6 diopters, 4.4 percent (2 of 44 eyes followed for one year) had lost two or more lines of best corrected acuity.[2] For higher myopes, 6 to 14 diopters, 7.6 percent (4 of 52 eyes) had lost two or more lines, after one year.[2] Of importance, eyes that were 20/20 with correction before surgery were no worse than 20/40 best corrected after LASIK.[2]

Another study directly compared PRK and LASIK in high myopia, 6 to 15 diopters in 220 eyes followed for six months.[3] Loss of best corrected vision was higher in the PRK treated patients than the LASIK ones. Haze which had not yet resolved in six months, however, may account for the difference.

9. Rise in Intraocular Pressure

Glaucoma is a condition in which the pressure in the eye rises high enough to cause damage to the optic nerve. The pressure at which damage occurs varies among individuals. Patients with pressures above 20 millimeters of mercury are observed for possible glaucoma. Use of steroid eye drops for more than ten to fourteen days will cause pressure rises in some people, who are referred to as "steroid responders." Discontinuing the steroid drops usually results in the pressure returning to baseline levels. Steroid drops are used in the post-operative management of PRK and LASIK patients, with longer use required for PRK.

In studying intraocular pressure rise in patients following PRK, 3.9 percent (19 of 542 eyes) were found to have increases of more than 5 millimeters of mercury, two years after the procedure.[1] Depending on their baseline intraocular pressure before surgery, and the ability of their optic nerve to withstand higher pressures, this may place them at higher risk for developing glaucoma. Intraocular pressure determination may be less accurate following LASIK or PRK.

10. Lens Abnormality

Clouding of the crystalline lens is referred to as a cataract. It is a natural occurrence with age. A lens abnormality was recorded in one of 520 eyes at one year after PRK for low to moderate myopia, and in three of 542 eyes followed two years after surgery.[1]

11. Ptosis

It is possible, though uncommon, to develop a droopy upper eyelid after laser vision correction. Use of a lid speculum, required for adequate exposure of the eye, can stretch or inflame the muscle responsible for raising and opening the eyelid. This can result in a droopy eyelid, causing the eye to appear "smaller." If this were to occur and not resolve on its own, it could be corrected with eyelid surgery.

12. Blindness

In surgery, as in life, anything is possible. Although there is not a reported case of permanent blindness occuring after PRK or LASIK surgery, it is a possibility. A serious infection inside the eye known as endophthalmitis could occur. Even with treatment it is possible that you could lose your eye. This very same problem could occur with contact lens wear if an ulcer progressed to endophthalmitis. Therefore, try to keep this fact in perspective.

The cornea could be damaged by the keratectomy during LASIK, or its surface made irregular enough by PRK or LASIK that your vision could be distorted to legal blindness levels. A cornea transplant, from a donor, could be required to replace the cornea. This operation should restore good vision, but healing from a transplant can take six to twelve months and rejection can occur, requiring repeat operations.

During certification courses for LASIK, physicians are usually shown a video of a disaster that occured in a case performed outside the U.S. The surgeon did not have the depth plate inserted in the microkeratome, and the eye was cut open under the high pressure created by the suction ring. The crystalline lens of the eye extruded. We are told that with corrective surgery the patient regained vision. Newer microkeratomes are designed to make this complication an impossibility.

The data presented on the loss of best corrected acuity should reassure you about the safety of laser vision correction.

Complications Due to the Keratectomy Step of the LASIK Procedure

All of the complications described above pertain to PRK and LASIK, although formation of haze is not an issue with the latter. There are complications that are specific to the keratectomy step and therefore are only a concern with LASIK. They include:

1. Incomplete Flap or Thin Flap

As described previously, the keratectomy is performed by an automated machine known as a microkeratome. It moves across a track on a suction ring, which generates high pressure in the eye to raise the dome of the cornea through its central opening.

If suction is lost before the keratectomy is completed, a thin flap will be created. The suction ring has a single hole through which the vacuum is created. If this becomes blocked or plugged, suction can be lost. If the surgeon moves the ring too much, suction can also be broken. A thin flap needs to be flipped back in position and allowed to heal. There are no reported cases where this has caused any permanent loss of vision. The keratectomy can be performed again after three months.

If the keratome is physically obstructed during its course along its track by eyelid tissue, plastic drape material or lid speculum, a partial flap will be created. This is more likely to occur in narrow eyes with deep set orbits where exposure is more difficult to achieve. The thickness of the cut will be fine, but it will not extend fully across the cornea as needed. This flap also needs to be repositioned and allowed to heal. The same outcome can occur if the surgeon takes his foot off the pedal and accidently replaces it on the wrong side of the pedal, which reverses the foward movement of the keratome. Again, this should all occur without visual consequence to the eye. There have been cases, however, where the surgeon has attempted to continue despite a partial flap, and decentered or incorrect treatments have resulted.

One LASIK study reported no thin caps in 404 eyes;[2] another study reported one incomplete and one thin flap in 220 surgeries.[3] The latter study reported that both of the patients were treated at a later date without complications.[3]

2. Damaged Microkeratome Blade

Any damage to the disposable microkeratome blade can create an irregular or torn flap. The part of the cutting surface that is unaffected will cut normally, but the nicked or damaged part of the blade will not. Prevention is the key through careful microscopic examination of the blade prior to surgery. A torn or irregular flap is allowed to heal and treatment delayed for three months.

There are a few frustrating stories about damaged blades that get aired at conferences. One university professor spoke of a blade which was inspected during keratome assembly but was damaged as the keratome rolled on the surgical tray before its use.

3. Flap Striae

Folds or wrinkles in the flap are known as **striae**. They disturb the smooth refractive surface of the cornea and thereby reduce vision. Any physical contact the eye undergoes, such as getting hit or rubbed, can displace the cap during the first few days after surgery.

In describing the LASIK procedure (pgs 48-53), it was noted that first the keratectomy is made, then the excimer laser treatment is applied, and finally the flap is floated back in place. On the first post-operative day, the cornea is checked carefully for any striae. If any are detected, the cap needs to be lifted and refloated in place, with gentle wiping to stretch out any folds. The longer that folds are allowed to remain in place, the harder it will be to remove them. However, they have been successfully removed even months after the intial procedure.

4. Free or Lost Cap

A free cap occurs during the keratectomy when the flap is cut completely across the cornea, leaving no connecting tissue. This can happen in eyes with flat corneas and in cases where the stop mechanism was not properly assembled. A free cap may dislodge after surgery and become lost, similar to a contact lens popping out.

LASIK was originally performed without a hinge and thus all flaps were "free." An experienced surgeon can anticipate and easily manage a free flap. Contrary to what one would expect, losing a flap is not a serious ordeal. Patients have been allowed to heal normally without the flap and have achieved excellent vision. The risk of developing haze is higher, however, particularly with deeper ablations.

One study reported no free flaps in 404 eyes treated by LASIK[2], another described one free cap in 220 eyes treated by LASIK.[3]

5. Epithelial Ingrowth

The corneal epithelium is not removed for the keratectomy as it is for PRK. However, the epithelium must be cut through by the keratome in order to get to the deeper stroma. It is possible for loosened epithelial cells to implant themselves beneath the flap. They can grow as a cluster or sheet of cells and multiply in the plane between the cap and the underlying stroma.

Sometimes the growth will be self-contained and remain near the outer perimeter of the flap. This is not a problem, but it needs to be observed closely because the growth can continue centrally toward the pupil. If this happens, vision would be disturbed and treatment would be required. The patient would be taken back to the laser suite or operating room to have the flap lifted. The epithelium would then be carefully scraped off the undersurface of the flap and the underlying stroma and the cap repositioned.

The incidence of epithelial ingrowth is about 2 percent, but most do not require treatment.[4] One study of 236 myopes, up to 6 diopters, reported a 1.7 percent incidence of epithelial ingrowth. Again, none required treatment.[2]

6. Infection

Surface ulceration and infection are less likely with LASIK than with PRK. However, infection can occur deeper in the cornea, beneath the flap. This area is closer to the inside of the eye, raising the risk of penetration of the infection into the eye. Therefore, infection needs to be treated aggressively. Any scarring can cause irregular healing in the overlying flap. Fortunately, occurrence is rare, about one in five thousand cases.

7. Sands of the Sahara (Diffuse Lamellar Keratitis)

Another complication involves a non-infectious infiltrate developing beneath the flap. A cloudy accumulation of inflammatory cells gives the appearance of swirling sand and has been dubbed "sands of the Sahara." The cause remains unclear. It has occurred in patients where the microkeratome is used to cut a flap, as well as in others where a previously cut flap was lifted for additional laser treatment. Only one eye of a patient who is treated bilaterally may be affected.

Sands of the Sahara is successfully treated by aggressively increasing the use of topical steroid eyedrops. The concern is to avoid any irregular healing in the flap. Severe cases may require lifting of the flap and removal of the inflammatory debris.

8. Irregular Astigmatism

Any of the above problems can contribute to the development of irregular astigmatism, see page 10. These complications can arise during the surgery or with post-operative healing and include: an uneven or irregular keratectomy; a decentered flap where the suction ring was not centered on the eye; a decentered ablation with the excimer laser; and problems with healing of the flap such as striae or wrinkles, epithelial ingrowth, infection, sands of the Sahara or loss of a free cap.

Any small irrgularities in how the flap lies back down on the underlying bed will affect the perfect smoothness of the surface. The more nearsighted you are, the more tissue that is removed by the laser. Perhaps the cap lies down less perfectly over the remodeled cornea.

Unlike regular astigmatism where the cornea is steeper in one axis, irregular astigmatism results from a variable unpredictable surface. Vision is reduced and can require a hard contact lens to achieve the best possible vision. The contact lens overlies the irregular surface and presents an artificially smooth one.

Most irregular astigmatism clears over the first month, but 1 or 2 percent of eyes have a significant residual irregular astigmatism that results in loss of best corrected visual acuity.

Eye Surgeons Who Have Had LASIK

The above laundry list of problems may seem intimidating to the prospective LASIK patient, and the potential risks do need to be considered. Perhaps the most impressive testimonial to the overall safety of the procedure comes from hundreds of ophthalmologists who have chosen to have LASIK performed on themselves.

In the RK era there were some eye surgeons who were patients also—who became "surgeons under the knife." The success of the laser procedures, PRK and LASIK, has led many more to have their vision corrected. These men and women who perform the procedures and know all the potential risks, are saying "yes" for themselves! That's an impressive vote of confidence for laser vision correction.

References

1. "VISX™ Excimer Laser System Photorefrative Keratectomy (PRK) Professional Use Information," copyright 1998, VISX Inc., Santa Clara, CA.

2. Lindstrom, R.; Hardten, D.; Chu, Y., Preschel, N.; and Jedicka, J., "Results of LASIK in 419 Eyes Using the VISX STAR Excimer Laser System," VISX, Inc., Santa Clara, CA.

3. Hersh, P.; Brint, S; Maloney, R; Durrie, D.; Gordon, M; Michelson, M; Thompson, V.; Berkeley, R.; Schein, O.; and Steinert, R.; "Photorefractive Keratectomy versus Laser In Situ Keratomileusis for Moderate to High Myopia — A Randomized Prospective Study," *Ophthalmology*, 1998; 105: 1512-1523.

4. Machat, Jeffery J.; *Excimer Laser Refractive Surgery — Practice and Principles*, Slack, Inc., NJ, 1996.

5
Can I Throw Away My Glasses or Contact Lenses?

Results of Laser Vision Correction

Results of PRK for Myopia and Astigmatism

We are now ready to discuss the results of excimer laser vision correction. Once again, the photorefractive keratectomy (PRK) data submitted by VISX to the FDA will be utilized.[1] Remember that we are discussing correcting distance vision. Reading vision is not treatable by the excimer laser, although one eye can be deliberately undercorrected to allow for near vision. If you are mildly nearsighted and able to read without glasses before laser surgery, you may require them for reading afterwards.

In the VISX data[1] there were 909 eyes treated by PRK with a 6 millimeter optical zone. Earlier work used smaller optical zones, which caused problems with night glare. When the data was submitted, 540 of these eyes had been followed for two years or longer. Sixty of them were eliminated from the analysis, 27 because they moved out of the area or were otherwise lost to follow up, and 33 who had a second treatment. Thus, the results with a single treatment on 480 eyes followed for at least two years will be summarized.

The patients were fairly evenly distributed across the range of myopia from 1 to 6 diopters:

-1 to -2	-2 to -3	-3 to -4	-4 to -5	-5 to -6
7.7%	15.6%	24.8%	26.7%	25.2%

Table 1
Results of PRK Treatment for Myopia Up to 6 Diopters

Uncorrected Visual Acuity *	Percent of 480 eyes
20/20 or better	58.3
20/25 to 20/40	35.8
20/50 to 20/80	5.8
20/100 or worse	.4

* vision without eyeglasses or contact lenses

Summarizing the results a little differently:

Table 2
Results of PRK Treatment for Myopia Up to 6 Diopters

Uncorrected Visual Acuity	Percent
20/20 or better	58
20/25 or better#	80
20/40 or better##	94

includes two groups of patients, those having 20/20 and 20/25 as their best visual acuity without glasses, respectively.

includes four groups of patients added together, those having 20/20, 20/25, 20/30, and 20/40 as their best visual acuity without glasses respectively.

Table 2 tells us that if you are a myope, up to 6 diopters, your chances of having 20/20 perfect distance vision without glasses is 58.3 percent with a single PRK treatment. Twenty-forty (20/40), the legal vision requirement for driving without glasses, was achieved by 94 percent of this group of patients, with a single treatment. Eighty percent were 20/25 or better. Remember that the smaller the denominator, the better the vision. Thus 20/25 is superior to 20/40. Refer to page 22.

Table 3
PRK Treatment for High Myopia 6 to 12 Diopters - Twelve Month Results

Uncorrected Visual Acuity	Percent
20/20 or better	50.6
20/30 or better#	80.1
20/40 or better ##	89.7

includes three groups of patients, those having 20/20, 20/25, and 20/30 as their best visual acuity without glasses, respectively.

includes four groups of patients added together, those having 20/20, 20/25, 20/30, and 20/40 as their best visual acuity without glasses respectively.

Results from VISX[2] on 200 eyes treated in Canada and the United Kingdom for high myopia, 6 to 12 diopters, and for astigmatism up to 4 diopters were slightly less than the lower degrees of myopia, but still quite impressive (table 3).

The speed at which vision is recovered following PRK is also important to examine. Of the group of 480 eyes shown in Table 4, uncorrected visual acuity improved over the first six months, with minimal change from six to twelve months, and then stability after that point.

Table 4
Uncorrected Visual Acuity As a Function of Time Since PRK Surgery for Myopia up to 6 Diopters[1]

Visual Acuity	Percent of Eyes at:					
	Prior to Surgery	1 Month	3 Months	6 Months	1 year	2 years
20/20 or better	0	32.3	45.5	55.8	63.7	58.3
20/25 to 20/40	0.4	57.3	47.5	38.7	31.4	35.4
20/50 to 20/80	5.0	9.2	46.7	5.5	4.7	5.8
20/100 or worse	94.6	1.1	0.7	0	0.3	0.4

Another way to analyze the success of PRK is to compare the results obtained to the correction entered into the laser. In other words, if a patient was -6 diopters, and full correction was selected in the computer, how close did the final refraction come to zero? In this same group of patients with up to 6 diopters of myopia, 65.5 percent were within 0.5 diopter, more or less, of the desired correction in a single treatment, and 90.2 percent within 1.0 diopter of intended correction.[1]

Can you throw away your glasses after laser vision correction? The answer depends, in part, upon you and your age. Millions of people walk around with 20/40 distance vision (or worse) and have never sought or accepted eyeglass correction for it. They function perfectly well for their own visual needs. However, people with poorer vision who have been used to wearing glasses or contacts most of their lives and have enjoyed the clarity of 20/20 vision, may be less tolerant of anything less than perfection. It is for these reasons that advertisements for laser vision correction will offer to "reduce or eliminate your need for eyeglasses or contact lenses." This means that you may get 20/20 without glasses and not need to wear them anymore, or you may get less than that but sufficient sight to not need glasses, or you may go without glasses for many activities but still use them for some.

Age is another factor that determines whether you can throw away your glasses. If you are in your late thirties to mid-forties you will need glasses to read if your myopia is corrected for distance.

Results of LASIK for Myopia and Astigmatism

As noted earlier, the FDA is still investigating the results of LASIK. Thus, there is no large-scale long time frame study to share with you as there is for PRK. LASIK has, however, shown similar results to PRK in smaller studies and has been performed in the United States since 1991.

Several private practice physicians have reported their results with LASIK in the medical literature. While these studies usually involve small numbers of patients, a few have large numbers. It takes a great deal of effort for a busy private practicioner to conduct a rigorous study. When the laser manufacturers sought FDA approval for their lasers for PRK, they dedicated a large support staff to track and organize the data.

Several studies are available on LASIK results. Some compile data from several surgeons operating at different centers. We will begin by summarizing some of the information in tables and will include PRK data for comparison.

Table 5
Uncorrected Visual Acuity Results for Treatment of Low to Moderate Myopia Up to 6 Diopters As a Function of Time Since Surgery — PRK versus LASIK

	Percent of Eyes at:			
	One Month		One Year	
Uncorrected Visual Acuity	PRK	LASIK	PRK	LASIK
	(n=436)	(n=231)	(n=344)	(n=44)
20/20 or better	32	69	64	64
20/25 or better	—	88	—	89
20/40 or better	90	97	95	96

n= shows the number of patients in each of the groups shown in the table column

PRK data from VISX, table 3-5 in PRK Professional Use Informational Manual [1]

— data not reported for 20/25 visual acuity level in this reference

LASIK data from Lindstrom, et. al. (reference # 3)

Table 5 shows us that vision improves more quickly with LASIK than with PRK. If you are a myope, up to 6 diopters, your chances of having 20/20 perfect distance vision without glasses, one month after surgery is 32 percent with PRK compared with 69 percent with LASIK. By one year, however, the results are almost identical. Sixty-four percent of myopic patients, up to 6 diopters treated by either PRK or LASIK, will have 20/20 vision without glasses and 95 percent will have 20/40 or better, which meets the standards for driving without glasses. LASIK and PRK results actually come very close to each other by three to six months in clinical practice.

Table 6
Uncorrected Visual Acuity Results for Treatment of High Myopia, Greater than 6 Diopters As a Function of Time Since Surgery — PRK versus LASIK

	Percent of Eyes at:			
	One Month		One Year	
	PRK	LASIK	PRK	LASIK
Uncorrected Vision		(n=144)	(n=156)	(n=44)
20/20 or better	—	36	51	40
20/25 or better	—	57	—	63
20/40 or better	—	86	90	84

PRK data from VISX, PRK Professional Use Informational Manual (reference # 2)

— data not reported at one month follow-up in reference # 2

LASIK data from Lindstrom, et. al. (reference #3)

Table 6 shows us that for both PRK and LASIK, the results are somewhat less effective for patients with myopia greater than 6 diopters. That is, a higher percentage of patients still needed glasses to see as well as the less near-sighted patients in Table 5. However, the percentage of patients achieving 20/40 or better is still quite impressive.

Comparing studies becomes difficult since the range of myopia treated varies, as does the period of time for patient follow-up. For example, in the PRK data shown in table 6, myopia from 6 to 12 diopters was treated, whereas in the LASIK data the upper limit extended to 15 diopters. This may explain the difference in results between the two procedures seen in Table 6. The difference is probably not statistically significant.

Another clinical trial evaluated the results of LASIK performed at twelve different centers on 202 eyes with myopia from as low as 1 diopter to as high as 10 diopters.[4] Data was for results six months from the time of surgery; longer follow-up was not reported. Sixty-eight percent were 20/20, 84 percent were 20/25 or better, and 93 percent were 20/40 or better. Loss of two or more lines of best corrected visual acuity occured in 2 eyes (1.5 percent). Ninety five percent of treated eyes were within 1 diopter of the intended result, and no eyes saw worse than 20/40 after surgery with correction by glasses or contact lenses.

One study compared PRK to LASIK for high myopia (6 to 15 diopters) by randomly assigning patients to receive one procedure or the other.[5] Data was combined on 220 eyes of 220 patients from seven clinical centers. This clinical trial confirmed the faster recovery of LASIK but the eventual similarity of results by three months. Results for uncorrected visual acuity were less impressive than the above reported studies. Post-operative results at six months from surgery included: 19.1 percent of the PRK eyes (n=68) were 20/20 without correction compared to 26.2 percent (n=61) of the LASIK eyes. Uncorrected visual acuity of 20/40 or better, (i.e. including 20/20, 20/25, 20/30 and 20/40), was reported in 66.2 percent of the PRK eyes, compared to 55.7 percent of the LASIK eyes. The difference, however, was not statistically significant.

None of the LASIK eyes developed corneal haze.[5] By six months 5.9 percent of the PRK eyes had mild (2+) haze and 4.4 percent had moderate (3+) haze. An interesting finding concerned loss of best corrected vision. At six months, 11.8 percent of the PRK treated eyes, compared to only 3.2 percent of the LASIK treated eyes had lost 2 or more lines of vision. Had the patients been followed longer, this difference may have gone away along with the haze.

Another study by Salah et. al., divided the results of LASIK by degree of myopia.[6] For 2 to 6 diopters 92.8 percent of patients achieved 20/40 or better uncorrected acuity. But for 6 to 12 diopters the percent, 20/40 or better uncorrected, dropped to 62.3 percent.

Results of PRK and LASIK for Hyperopia

FDA approval of PRK for hyperopia was first granted to VISX, on November 2, 1998. Thus, compared with myopia and astigmatism, there are far fewer studies, with smaller numbers of patients and shorter periods of patient follow up. Most of the information comes from abroad and from U.S. clinical trials performed for FDA approval.

In the data supplied to the FDA by VISX, 124 eyes of 124 patients were treated at several centers in the U.S. and 42 eyes in Canada. All patients were followed for at least one year.[7]

Table 7
Uncorrected Visual Acuity Following PRK for Hyperopia

Visual Acuity	1 Month (n=166)	6 Months (n=150)	1 Year (n=97)
% 20/20 or better	13.3	53.3	63.9
% 20/25 or better #	26.5	73.3	80.4
% 20/40 or better ##	60.2	96.0	94.8

n= shows the number of patients in each of the groups shown in the table column

includes two subgroups of patients: those who were able to see the 20/20 line without glasses and those who read the 20/25 line as their best vision without glasses.

includes four subgroups of patients added together, those having 20/20, 20/25, 20/30, and 20/40 as their best visual acuity without glasses respectively.

At one year 75.7 percent of treated eyes were within 0.5 diopters of the intended correction and 92.2 percent were within one diopter.[7]

The results of PRK for hyperopia are quite impressive. LASIK for hyperopia is showing faster visual rehabilitation than PRK, with otherwise similar long term outcomes. LASIK and PRK for hyperopia both have an initial over-correction to nearsightedness. This gradually fades over 6 months toward no refractive error.

Conclusion

It is the speed of recovery and the comfort during the early post-operative period that is driving the growing popularity of LASIK over PRK, not the long term results. LASIK is also easier to enhance or add correction to if needed, and lacks the problem of haze.

One study illustrates the point about recovery time. Patients received either LASIK or PRK for treatment of their first eye and the opposite procedure for their second eye.[8] Those receiving PRK requested the "better laser" they had heard about from other patients in the waiting room, referring to the ones treated by LASIK. Despite patient preference for LASIK, this study also showed similar long-term improvement in vision for both procedures.

References

1. VISX™ Excimer Laser System—Photorefractive Keratectomy (PRK) Professional Use Information, copyright 1998, VISX Inc., Santa Clara, CA.

2. *Physician's Training Manual for VISX Excimer Laser System,* section on "Photorefractive Keratectomy for High Myopia with Astigmatism," copyright 1998, Visx, Inc., Santa Clara, CA.

3. Lindstrom, L.; Hardten, D.; Chu, Y.; Preschel, N.; and Jedicka, J.; *Results of LASIK in 419 Eyes Using the VISX Star Excimer Laser System,* copyright 1998, VISX, Inc.

4. Lindstrom, R., *The Barraquer Lecture: Surgical Management of Myopia – A Clinician's Perspective,* J.Refractive Surg., 13: 287- 294, 1997.

5. Hersh, P.; Brint, S.; Maloney, R.; Durrie, D.; Gordon, M.; Michelson, M.; Thompson,V.; Bekeley, R.; Schein, O.; Steinert, R.; "Photorefractive Keratectomy versus Laser In Situ Keratomileusis for Moderate to High Myopia," *Ophthalmology* 1998; 105: 1512-1523.

6. Salah T., Waring G., El-Maghraby A., et al. "Excimer Laser in Situ Keratomileusis under a Corneal Flap for Myopia of 2 to 20 Diopters." Am J. Ophthalmol 1996; 121:143-155.

7. VISX STAR S2 Excimer Laser System Photorefractive Keratectomy (PRK) Professional Use Information, pgs. 32-36, VISX, Inc., Santa Clara, CA.

8. Steven Slade, M.D. Personal communication.

6
What's in the Future? Should I Wait?

$\mathcal{T}$ here are many questions to ponder in deciding whether or not to undergo laser vision correction. Preceeding chapters have addressed safety and success. Cost will be covered later. The next important questions are: *Should I wait? Is there something better coming in the future?* There are other procedures in an evaluation stage and these will be discussed here, in addition to a related question: *will laser vision correction improve?*

There are two considerations for determining whether you should wait:

1. Is the present LASIK or PRK procedure already good enough to satisfy your needs?

2. How much time are you willing to wait?

Once we reach our thirties we begin to realize how quickly life passes. You want to enjoy freedom or at least significantly less dependence on glasses or contact lenses. How much more time do you want to let pass, worrying that something better may be coming? In evaluating the risks and benefits of alternative procedures to reduce the need for eyeglasses or contact lenses, there is nothing that has yet proven to be superior to laser vision correction.

Alternatives to Laser Vision Correction— Non-surgical

Eyeglasses and contact lenses are two obvious, non-surgical alternatives to laser vision correction. Eyeglasses are safe as long as they don't get knocked off your face, stepped on during an emergency, or steamed up with temperature changes to blur your vision. They are of no help when swimming in a pool and are at risk in many recreational activities, such as water or snow skiing, or jogging in the rain. On the plus side, they serve as a barrier to objects hitting your eyes, as long as the lenses are shatterproof.

Contact lenses are not as safe as might be assumed. Few people consider the risks involved, particularly with an infection, known as a **corneal ulcer**. When ulcers heal, they leave a scar. If the scar is over the center of your cornea, your vision may be significantly reduced. Some patients have required corneal transplant surgery following contact lens related corneal ulcers (figure 36 A and B).

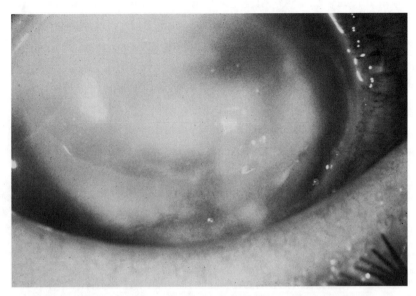

Figure 36A—Severe contact lens related corneal ulcer

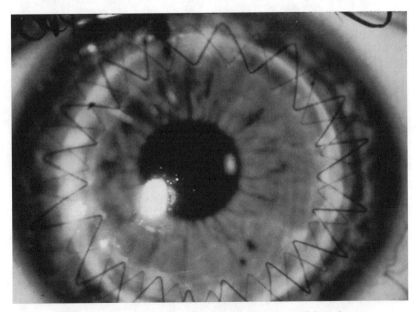

Figure 36B—Cornea transplant sutured in place

The key to avoiding complications is prevention. Extended wear contact lenses, the ones that you sleep with, put you at higher risk of developing an infection. It's safer to remove and clean your lenses each night. If your eye gets red and irritated when wearing a contact lens, remove it. If the redness and irritation doesn't go away in a few hours, see your eye doctor. Patients who follow these precautions may develop an ulcer, but almost all will recover well with treatment. It's important that you have a spare pair of glasses to wear, with an up-to-date prescription, for times when you are unable to wear your lenses.

A less recognized risk from contact lenses is penetration of the eye by fragments of hard or gas permeable lenses with blunt trauma. Fortunately, this is uncommon. More typical problems with contact lenses involve external irritation and inflammation of the eye. Many people have dry eyes and keeping their contacts moist is a problem. When contact lenses become dry, a person's vision becomes blurry and his eyes red and irritated. Common aggravants for these patients are air conditioning, a breeze from an open window or fan, cigarette smoke, and air travel.

Allergies are another major problem for contact lens patients. Protein build up from the tear film and mucous can deposit on the lenses. This reduces comfort and vision, explaining the popularity of disposable lenses. Some patients actually develop allergic reactions to this debris. Chemicals, particularly preservatives in the cleaning solutions, are another common allergen. The result is uncomfortable contact lens wear with red, watery, itchy eyes and reduced vision. Prescription eye drops may help reduce the symptoms, but many of these patients will ultimately discontinue contact lens wear.

Surgical Alternatives to Contact Lens Wear

Intraocular Contact Lens or Phakic Intraocular Lens

As mentioned in chapter one, there are two lenses that focus light in the eye (see figure 1). The first is the corneal lens and the second the crystalline lens. By making changes in the power of either lens, refractive errors can be corrected. While laser vision correction changes the cornea, intraocular lenses add to the power of the crystalline lens or replace it.

If the crystalline lens becomes cloudy with age, it can be removed. This is known as cataract surgery. Years ago, cataracts were removed without replacing the lens, leaving the eye "**aphakic**." Patients were left to suffer with extremely thick glasses or were given contact lenses to correct their vision. The improvement of the intraocular lens, or IOL, is a major advance of the last twenty years. By measuring the length of the eye and the curvature of the cornea, a computer is able to estimate the proper IOL power to correct a patient's vision. The length of the eye is measured by an ultrasound probe held up against the cornea—a procedure similar to obtaining pictures of a baby in the mother's womb.

The cloudy crystalline lens (cataract) has a clear outer capsule. During the removal surgery, which uses ultrasonic vibrations of a needle, not laser, most of the capsule is left in place to support the small plastic IOL. The eye is then said to be **"pseudophakic,"** or to have a false (pseudo) lens (phakia).

From the standpoint of correcting a refractive error, IOLs are a successful modality. More than a million seniors each year, following cataract surgery, enjoy better vision without glasses than ever before in their lives. For a younger patient, however, whose crystalline lens is not cloudy, there is an important disadvantage to removing it. Accommodation (the ability of the human lens to change focus from far to near and vice versa) is lost. Some research is on-going to develop a liquid plastic that could be injected into the empty capsular bag, which might possibly allow accommodation to continue. This work is probably still many years from human clinical trials, but it's an interesting idea.

What to do for the younger person with a clear crystalline lens, the **"phakic"** patient who wants to see without eyeglasses, remains a question. One answer lies in leaving the natural lens in place and inserting a plastic intraocular lens in front of the crystalline lens. We refer to this lens as a **Phakic IOL** or **Intraocular Contact Lens**. The IOL and the human lens in combination with the cornea would then focus light and correct for refractive errors.

Three main advantages are present for this approach compared with PRK and LASIK. The first one is the reversible nature of the surgery. If the lens causes problems for any reason—haloes, glare, incorrect power—it can be removed. Second, the normal contour of the corneal surface is not disturbed. Third, there is no diopter limit to the correction of myopia or hyperopia.

On the downside are some serious potential complications that need to be considered. These will be discussed below. Also, while phakic IOLs are available to correct myopia and hyperopia, there is none that can also correct astigmatism. Thus, a separate procedure would be required to correct significant amounts of astigmatism, such as an astigmatic keratotomy (AK), see pg 36, or laser vision correction.

There are three styles of phakic IOLs presently in evaluation by the FDA. Two sit "anterior" or in front of the iris or pupil, and one sits "posterior" or behind the pupil, but in front of the crystalline lens. One of the anterior style lenses has feet which anchor into the wall of the eye (figure 37), and the other has two claws which clip on to the iris or colored part of the eye (figure 38).

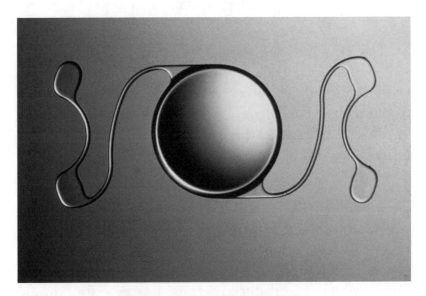

Figure 37—NuVita Phakic IOL
Courtesy of Bausch & Lomb Surgical

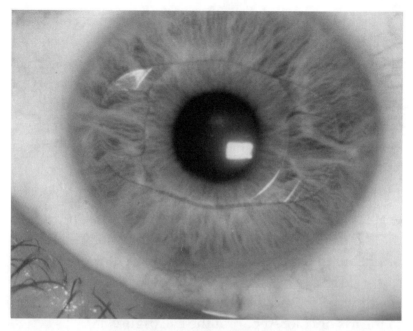

Figure 38—Artisan Myopia Lens
Courtesy of Ophtec

The two anterior lenses are made of polymethyl-methacrylate or PMMA, similar to plexiglass, and the posterior "implantable contact lens" is made of a mixture of soft materials, collagen and hydrogel. This soft lens can be folded and inserted through a smaller incision than the others. Regardless of the lens type, the placement and positioning inside the eye creates complications that have been observed, and others which remain a concern.

To understand one important complication, we first need to discuss **intraocular pressure** or "**IOP**." The human eye continually makes a salty fluid called "**aqueous humor**," which is produced inside the eye and drains through the "angle" of the eye (figure 39). The eye "pressure" or IOP is a balance of the amount of fluid produced in the eye versus the amount drained. The drain is comprised of a sieve-like structure called the trabecular meshwork. As we age, it sometimes functions less efficiently, leading to a condition known as **glaucoma**, where the pressure in the eye rises to abnormal levels. High IOP can damage the optic nerve in the back of the eye, initially causing a loss of peripheral vision followed by central vision loss if left untreated. Since we cannot feel pain or pressure when our IOP is elevated, routine eye exams are recommended.

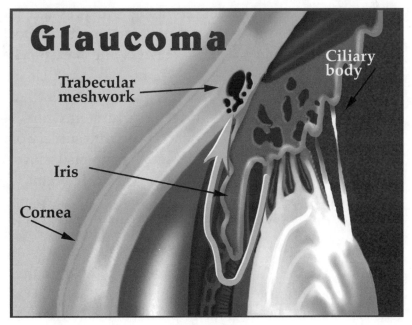

Figure 39

As mentioned above, the placement of phakic IOLs leads to several possible complications. One is the creation of elevated IOP or glaucoma. One style of anterior phakic IOL has plastic feet that anchor into the "angle," near, but not in, the trabecular meshwork (figure 37). This placement is not easy to perform initially, and the lenses may shift position after surgery. The foot plate of the lens can entangle in the iris and distort the pupil or lead to scarring in the angle with blockage of the drain. In a recent published report from France on this style lens, 30 of 133 eyes, (27.8 percent) had iris retraction and ovalization of the pupil from this very process.[1] This was reported as generally of no clinical significance. Despite these changes, only 1 of 90 eyes (1.1 percent) at one year, and 0 of 37 eyes followed for three years, had an abnormal eye pressure.[1]

Another mechanism for elevating eye pressure is blockage of the pupil by the IOL, obstructing the flow of aqueous from behind it. This is known as **pupillary block glaucoma**. It can usually be avoided by making a hole in the peripheral iris, creating another path for the fluid to drain out. This opening is known as an **iridectomy**, and it can be accomplished with a laser days prior to surgery or at the time of IOL insertion. In the study mentioned above, iridectomies were not done on all patients, only on those "presumed to be at risk."[1] The authors did not explain how they determined their selection. Four eyes (3.0 percent) developed pupillary block.

A study from Argentina reported on 124 eyes that received the soft, foldable intraocular contact lens.[2] This lens is placed posterior to the pupil. Six of the eyes developed pupillary block. Four of these did not have an iridectomy. Two did, but it was no longer open. Another concern with this style of lens is development of a cataract from contact of the IOL with the crystalline lens. Only one eye (0.9 percent) formed a cataract, and it resulted from the preoperative iridectomy.[2] There was one eye excluded from the study because the phakic IOL hit the crystalline lens during positioning and resulted in a cataract. There were no other IOL-induced cataracts in this series.

One concern for all three styles of phakic IOLs is damage to the innermost lining of the cornea, the endothelial cell layer. The cornea, which sits bathed in the aqueous humor, is able to avoid swelling, thereby maintaining its clarity by the activity of these cells. As fluid enters the endothelial cells, they are capable of pumping it back out. Endothelial cells are not able to multiply. Therefore, once damaged they cannot be replaced. Some are gradually lost due to age. During surgery, with insertion of the IOL, the corneal endothelial cells can be touched and damaged. After surgery, rubbing of the eye can put the IOL in contact with the back surface of the cornea. This can occur during sleep when the patient is unaware of his action. In one study of an anterior phakic IOL, endothelial cell loss was 3.3 percent at six months, with an additional loss of 1 to 2 percent over the remaining two and a half years of follow-up.[1] This is a minimal amount that would not cause problems. Other studies have reported greater losses of 12 to 18 percent with an anterior phakic IOL model.[3] This would be tolerated by a young patient without corneal swelling. Over time, however, if endothelial damage were progressive, it could cause corneal edema and reduced vision.

Other complications with phakic IOLs include haloes and glare. In one study these symptoms were reported in 27.8 percent of patients, declining to 12.5 percent at three years.[1] The lens diameter was only 4 millimeters. As explained earlier this is not a large enough optical zone to focus light when the pupil dilates at night. Another risk is infection. Since the eye is opened with an incision to insert the lens, the possibility of germs getting direct access into the eye exists, as it does with cataract surgery. Although the incidence of serious infection with cataract surgery is only one in a thousand or more cases, there can be permanent serious loss of vision. In some patients, another problem with IOLs is chronic inflammation of the eye by the foreign plastic material.

At the present time phakic IOLs are under FDA investigation. There are published reports from around the world, as mentioned above. These studies included extremely nearsighted patients, from -7 up to -18.80 diopters[1] and -8.50 to -18.63 diopters.[2] The upper ranges of myopia include many patients whose vision is below normal. As an example, of the 134 eyes in one study, only 80 percent, could see 20/40 or better with correction before surgery.[2] Thus, it is not relevant to compare the percent of eyes after surgery that could see 20/40 or better without correction to the PRK data where all eyes had normal vision before surgery. Only 52.9 percent of 70 eyes given a phakic IOL were 20/40 or better without correction at two years after surgery.[1] For comparison, the post-operative uncorrected visual acuity for PRK can be found in Table 3, pg. 83. It should be noted that the PRK data represents myopes up to twelve diopters, a much easier group to correct.

We can, however, compare how close to zero refractive error the eyes were following surgery. In the posterior phakic intraocular lens study, 86 eyes (69 percent) were within 1 diopter of intended correction, under or overcorrected from the zero target point, and 55 eyes (44 percent) were within the tighter range of +/_ 0.5 diopter.[2] In the anterior phakic IOL study, 69.1 percent of 68 eyes were

within +/– 1.0 diopter, and 41.2 percent were within +/–
0.5 diopters.[1]

In summary, phakic intraocular lenses present an in-
triguing alternative to laser vision correction. The strong
points include:

1.   Ability for high corrections beyond the limit of LASIK
      and PRK

2.   Reversibility

3.   Lack of change to the surface of the cornea

4.   Familiarity to eye surgeons of working with IOLs

Most eye surgeons are very comfortable with IOLs,
since cataract surgery traditionally represents the most
common procedure performed in their practices. The accuracy of predicting phakic IOL lens power will need to
be refined. As the number of surgeries performed increases, phakic IOLs should produce visual results equal
to or better than LASIK for patients not requiring astigmatism correction. In fact, a few surgeons outside the U.S.
have implanted a phakic IOL in one eye and performed
LASIK in the patient's fellow eye. Reportedly, some patients express a preference for the vision in the eye with
the IOL.[4]

On the downside are an assortment of complications
which have been explained above. These are serious
enough to cause many U.S. surgeons to heavily weigh the
decision to consider a phakic IOL. With laser vision cor-

rection as accurate and safe as it has shown to be, IOLs will probably take a back seat to the excimer laser for low to moderate myopes. In addition, the inability to correct astigmatism with phakic IOLs remains a major problem. Improved lens designs may change the situation. A growing interest, however, is being expressed for using this technology for the higher ranges of myopia and hyperopia, where LASIK and PRK fail. This limit, for LASIK, is somewhere in the vicinity of -12 diopters of myopia, and + 6 diopters of hyperopia. For these groups of patients, phakic IOLs may hold the best promise.

Intrastromal Corneal Ring Segments (Intacs™)

Another alternative to laser vision correction is the use of the **intrastromal corneal ring segments (ICRS)**, (figure 40). Two curved segments are placed in the cornea through a small incision, each measures 150 degrees of arc. These segments are able to flatten the cornea and reduce myopia. In this procedure, myopia correction is FDA approved from -1.00 to -3.00 diopters. While no correction for astigmatism is yet available, it may be possible to use two different ring segments to correct the unequal curvature. The ring segments are approved in Canada for treatment of myopia from -1 to -5 diopters.

The main appeal of the ICRS is the reversibility of the procedure, since the segments can be removed. Reasons for removal have included undercorrection, overcorrection, astigmatism created by the forces of the ring segments (induced astigmatism), glare, fluctuation of vision and Staphylococcus aureus infection.[5, 6] Corneal topography returns to pre-operative status within three months of removal.

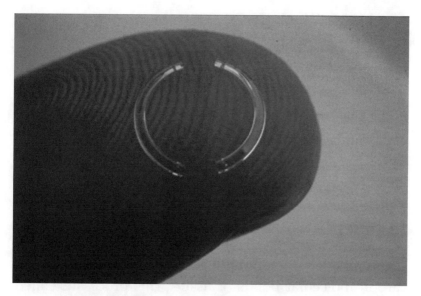

Figure 40—Intrastromal corneal ring segments
Photo courtesy Keravision, Inc.

Intrastromal corneal ring segments at present are a limited weapon in the artillery against refractive errors. The range of myopia correction is limited, and hyperopia and astigmatism are not yet treatable. Future developments need to be watched.

Future Improvements to Laser Vision Correction

Lasers are computer driven instruments, and as such we are likely to see improvements in software and hardware. The U.S. tends to lag behind the rest of the world because of slow FDA approval. Thus, for a glimpse into the future, one does not need a crystal ball but only to look at other countries to see what new developments are coming or are already in use.

The Magic Black Box

Excimer lasers are big, impressive machines with fancy control panels. In order to appreciate the differences between machines, you need to understand some basic design.

The laser head is the main section and consists of a gas cavity and electrodes. Argon and flouride gases are mixed to fill the cavity. Electricity is then used to "excite" the gases to higher energy states causing the release of ultraviolet light energy, wavelength 193 nanometers. Because two gases are excited in the process, the term "**excimer**" was coined, for excited dimer. The far ultraviolet light energy that is released is strong enough to break down the carbon-carbon molecular bonds of tissue. This process is called photoablative decomposition of tissue or "photoablation."

The laser cavity contains mirrors (figure 41). One reflects the light back and forth to continue the reaction described above. Another allows some light to be transmitted to the delivery portion of the laser. The transmitted light travels through lenses and is bent and reflected by mirrors and prisms, until it reaches a diaphragm. By controlling the size, pattern and duration of the diaphragm opening, the treatment can be controlled. Thus, for astigmatism, one axis of the cornea is treated more than the other by varying how much of the diaphragm is open and at what axis.

The laser light loses some of its energy as it travels through the machine. It can also damage the delicate mirrors and lenses. During calibration of the laser, testing needs to be done to confirm that the laser beam is delivering the intended output. The laser light beam should be homogenous, with equal energy distributed across its diameter. Damage to mirrors and optical lenses can create beams with "**cold spots**," where energy is weaker than the surrounding beam, or "**hot spots**," where energy is higher. During PRK or LASIK, instead of creating an even ablation of the corneal tissue, these cold or hot spots would cause less or more of the corneal tissue to be ablated than intended.

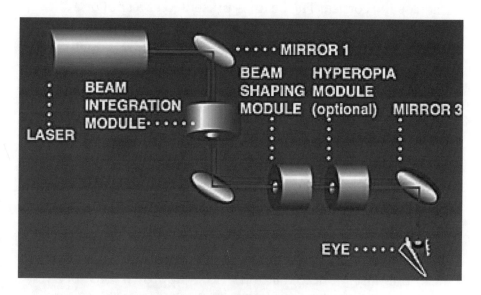

Figure 41—Schematic of excimer laser
Courtesy of VISX, Inc.

Scanning Versus Broad Beam Lasers

We are now in a position to understand some of the differences between lasers. The first two lasers approved for use in the U.S., VISX and Summit, are "**broad beam lasers**." This means that the beam size equals the entire diameter of the treatment. Thus, the beam diameter is 6 millimeters, which is the size of the treatment zone of a PRK. For a myopic treatment without astigmatism, the laser fires successive pulses with the treatment zone expanding up to 6 millimeters as the iris diaphragm gradually opens to full diameter. VISX has since modified its technology. (see below)

A **scanning or "flying spot" laser**, in contrast, uses a smaller diameter laser beam, one to two millimeters, and rotating optics to fire the beam in an organized pattern across the cornea. The beam is presented as a spot or a slit which is scanned over the cornea in an overlapping fashion to create a smooth contour. Manufacturers include Chiron Technolas (flying spot), CIBA-Autonomous Technologies (flying spot), Nidek (scanning slit) and Aesculap-Meditec(scanning slit). Advantages claimed for the scanning lasers include ease of maintaining a homogenous beam because its diameter is smaller, a smoother treatment surface, and a smaller acoustic shock wave that is gentler on the cornea. Smoothness is more important for the surface treatment of PRK than in LASIK, where the treated cornea is covered by the cap. LASIK success is 90 percent dependent on a good keratectomy and 10 percent on the laser photoablation. FDA approval has been granted for Autonomous Technologies and for Nidek. Time will tell if we can perceive a difference in results compared to broad beam lasers.

VISX has already introduced a modification to smooth the ablation contour, called VISX SmoothScan™. This is featured in their STAR 2 (S2) laser. A single broad beam is split into seven beams, that rotate when the laser is in use. This creates a hybrid scanning-broad beam laser. The diameter of the overall ablation increases from two to six millimeters for myopic corrections, as the diameter of the constituent beams gradually enlarges and their overlap of one another becomes greater.

Eye Trackers

As explained earlier, during the laser treatment you fixate on a red light. The surgeon observes your fixation through a microscope with an overlying reticule to determine that the treatment is centered on your eye. If there is eye movement the surgeon lifts his foot from the laser pedal and the procedure is temporarily stopped. When you regain fixation, the procedure resumes. Since the treatment only takes between 30 to 90 seconds, this happens rarely, if at all.

There is another, more high tech solution to the issue of fixation. The laser can track your eye movements. This process has been developed by Autonomous Technologies and Chiron-Technolas.

A "passive" tracker would turn the laser off if you moved your eye too far from the fixation light. An "active" eye tracker, as developed by Autonomous Technologies and Chiron-Technolas, enables the laser to move in synchronization with any movement of your eye while continuing the treatment. Although it sounds good, it's uncertain whether eye-tracking will make a difference in clinical results compared to a broad beam laser without a tracker. Autonomous uses a small scanning spot, less than one millimeter in diameter and Chiron-Technolas uses a two millimeter spot. Since these lasers fire a pattern of small spots on the cornea, the placement is more critical than with a wide beam which covers the full six millimeter optical zone. Scanning lasers, therefore, are less forgiving of small eye movement and more dependent on a tracker than are the broad beam lasers such as VISX and Summit.

In November, 1998, Autonomous received FDA approval for PRK from one to ten diopters, with or without astigmatism up to four diopters. Chiron-Technolas awaits FDA approval.

Corneal Topography Assisted Laser Ablations

Perhaps the most promising research is the use of real time corneal topography to guide the laser ablation. Imagine if the laser could ablate a map of your specific corneal shape, rather than a generic pattern. The topography would be "on-line" with the laser treatment, guiding the ablation until the desired affect was accomplished. Currently, if a patient has astigmatism that is steeper vertically, the present laser technology will apply more treatment to this axis. However, many patients are not uniformly steep across an axis (figure 42). A better result for the patient

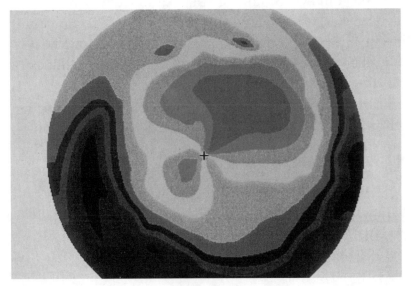

Figure 42

shown in figure 42 would occur if more ablation were applied to the upper half of the vertical axis, where the cornea is asymmetrically steeper.

There is now a limited capabilility for doing topography guided treatment "off-line." If a patient has a decentered treatment, the laser company can pre-program an ablation pattern onto a card. That card is inserted into the laser which then customizes the ablation.

Automatic Refraction Guided Laser Ablation

Instead of using a map of the corneal surface to guide the treatment, a machine which measures the patient's refractive error could be "on-line" and guide the ablation until the refractive error is reduced to zero. "Autorefractors" have been used in eye doctors' offices for years to determine a patient's eyeglass prescription.

Computerized feedback from a light that first passes through the cornea, then the crystalline lens, and finally focuses on the retina, would be used to adjust the laser treatment.

Microkeratomes

The instrument used to create the corneal flap may see improvements in design. Most of the cases in the U.S. and around the world have been performed with the Chiron Automatic Corneal Shaper (ACS) unit, shown in figure 29. The ACS unit was conceived nearly a decade ago, and was used in refractive procedures that preceeded the excimer laser and LASIK. Chiron is now producing a newer model, the Hansatome, and is joined in the field by eighteen other manufacturers. Features that vary among the units are: the speed of oscillation of the blade; the type of blade; the power source, electric versus gas turbine; and the cutting head, disposable versus reusable. The Chiron ACS unit uses an electric motor which drives its gears and oscillates a disposable stainless steel blade at 8,000 times per minute as it cuts through the corneal tissue.

Some of the other units use a gas turbine power source that is capable of oscillating the blade at frequencies up to 20,000 times per minute. The significance of the oscillation rate is that the faster the oscillation, the smoother the cut that can be produced. This may have clinical significance, but it has not been reported.

Another option is the material used for the cutting blade, which is usually stainless steel. In some models the option of a reusable diamond or sapphire blade is given. Again, a gem quality blade should be capable of a smoother cut, but small nicks in the re-usable cutting surface might be a concern. Neither of the Chiron units allows the surgeon to visualize the flap as it is being cut. Several other manufacturers have created a clear window through which the surgeon can watch as the flap is made.

Finally, other modalities than blades are being investigated for cutting the flap. A high power jet stream of water is one consideration and a laser light a second. As you can tell, this is a fast moving, exciting field.

In summary, the remarks made in the beginning of the chapter deserve repeating: You need to decide if laser vision correction is a good choice for you. If so, with the results for PRK and LASIK as good as they are already, do you want to sit around worrying that something better may become available down the road? If you're ready to do something about your vision, go for it.

References

1. Baikoff, G.; et al. "Angle-fixated Anterior Chamber Phakic Intraocular Lens for Myopia of -7 to -19 Diopters," *Journal of Refractive Surgery*, 1998, 14:282-293.

2. Zaldivar, R.; Davidorf, J.; Oscherow, S. "Posterior Chamber Phakic Intraocular Lens for Myopia of -8 to -19 Diopters, *Journal of Refractive Surgery*, 1998, 14:294-305.

3. Perez-Santonja, J.; Iradier, M.; Sanz-Iglesias, L.; Serrano, J.; Zato, M. "Endothelial changes in phakic eyes with anterior chamber intraocular lenses to correct high myopia." *Journal of Cataract Refractive Surgery*, 1996; 22:1017-1022.

4. Monroe, L., "Phakic IOLs — The Future of Refractive Surgery?" *EyeNet*, August 1998: 20-21, American Academy of Ophthalmology.

5. Surgeon Gives Advice on Performing ICRS Explantation, *Ocular Surgery News*, 1998, 16(15):54-55, Slack, NJ.

6. Richard Abbott, M.D., personal communication.

7
Why Don't All Eye Doctors Recommend Laser Vision Correction?

*B*y now a great deal of information has been presented to you about laser vision correction. You're probably trying to decide whether or not to undergo the procedure. It's time to turn to your family and friends, to your common sense, to patients who have had the procedure and perhaps to another medical professional. Research has shown that many people consult their regular eye doctor for laser vision correction, and for most patients that is not the ophthalmologist who will be doing the procedure.

It turns out that many people who are candidates for laser vision correction see optometrists and not ophthalmologists. Don't feel ignorant if you don't know the difference. Studies have shown that half of the population does not. An optometrist is a doctor of optometry and holds an O.D. degree. This degree is obtained after four years of study in optometry school, which follows college. An optometrist is not licensed to perform surgery, but is allowed in most states to treat medical eye problems with eye drops.

An ophthalmologist holds an M.D. degree, granted after four years of medical school, similar to your family doctor, pediatrician or gynecologist. He or she then serves an internship in internal medicine or general surgery and then completes a minimum of three years of residency training in eye surgery and management of eye diseases.

If you ask your eye doctor whether laser vision correction is a good idea for you, don't be surprised if the response is negative even though you may be an excellent candidate. Since this book is a consumer's guide, we need to speak honestly about the reasons for this. Factors that may lead to a negative response include:

1. Lack of knowledge or experience with laser vision correction

2. Anticipated loss of income from not selling you contact lenses and eyeglasses

3. Fear of losing your ongoing care to the laser surgeon

4. Prior negative experience with RK or other refractive procedure

5. Conservative approach toward surgery in general

Try to put yourself in the position of your optometrist, or an ophthalmologist who has not yet trained in PRK or LASIK, when you inquire about laser vision correction. Optometrists derive their income from performing eye exams and selling contact lenses and glasses. The possibility of hundreds of thousands, perhaps even a million patients undergoing laser vision correction each year is viewed by them as a threat to their profession. Their reaction is understandably negative. It's hard to remain objective. In reality, the threat is not so great. Millions of myopes will never desire or choose to spend their money on laser vision correction regardless of how good it is. Many of those that do, including the baby boomers, will still need reading glasses. (Of course, these could be inexpensive store-bought reading glasses for many after laser vision correction.) Some laser vision correction patients will still want weak eyeglass prescriptions to provide 20/20 vision, if LASIK or PRK did not provide that level of visual acuity. Finally, quality sunglasses will be desired as well. Laser patients get excited about their opportunity to wear those non-prescription sunglasses that always look so great on other people.

If your regular eye doctor is not the ophthalmologist who would be performing the laser surgery, there is likely to be some concern on his part that you may wish to stay under the care of the laser surgeon. The reality is that the laser surgeon probably does not wish to interfere with your established relationship.

After your post-operative care is completed, he would probably prefer to make room in his practice for the next group of laser patients. In some cases, your post-operative care may be performed in whole or part by your regular eye doctor (see page 129). However, it's important for you to understand how your interest in seeking care elsewhere for laser vision correction may be threatening to your regular provider.

Your optometrist's prior experiences with refractive surgery is another important variable. He may never have managed any patients who have had refractive surgery. Worse yet, he may have had a patient who had less than an ideal result with RK. Or he may have heard stories from colleagues that have given him a sour outlook. Laser vision correction is still new enough that many eye doctors may not have yet followed one of their own patients through it.

Finally, optometrists tend to be conservative in general when it comes to surgery. That's not a bad thing. It's good to have balance, to look with a cautious eye toward any type of elective surgery, including laser vision correction. He may be of the opinion that as long as you can see with glasses, why take any risks?

On the other hand, many optometrists are jumping on the laser vision correction bandwagon, and many have themselves had the procedure. They have been impressed by the results and are participating in the management of their patients after surgery and beyond. This group of proactive optometrists are readily encouraging their patients who have difficulty with contact lenses to consider laser vision correction.

The preceding discussion is not meant to denigrate the motives behind all doctors who speak against these procedures. Some do so with a pure heart, entirely in your interest. For others, it's a mixture of selfish and genuine professional concerns. What's important is that you maintain an open mind and listen to all viewpoints but be skeptical about the motives behind any negative criticism you hear.

8
Why Does it Cost So Much?

The Business Side of Laser Vision Correction

*N*o consumer's guide would be complete without some discussion of finances. Laser vision correction is costly to undergo as a patient, and to provide as a surgeon. We'll examine the factors involved and try to leave you with a better understanding of why it costs what it does, and if that's likely to change soon.

Several of the expenses that will be discussed are not charged directly to the patient. They are paid by whomever owns or leases the laser. As such, these expenses reduce the profit margin, and can run a laser vision correction practice in debt for some time. Ophthalmologists typically use the income from their existing cataract practices to offset the losses incurred in establishing a laser vision correction practice. Laser vision correction is not the "cash cow" that it may seem to you, as you wait your turn on a surgery day and count the number of patients.

It is hoped that the detailed description of PRK (pages 38-43) and LASIK (pages 48-53) will give the reader an appreciation of the skill involved, particularly in performing the keratectomy. Unlike PRK whose success is mostly dependent on the laser, LASIK is heavily dependent on the skill of the surgeon. Caveat emptor — buyer beware. Please don't look for a bargain because it only takes twenty minutes. The surgeon's heart and every ounce of his concentration and fine motor skills are focused on you. His talents will bring you a lifetime of freedom to enjoy seeing the world around you.

Finally, financing plans are available to make laser vision correction affordable for everyone.

The Laser

The greatest expense is the laser. This is probably not a surprise to you. The two lasers in common use in the U.S., VISX and Summit, cost about half a million dollars to purchase. Most eye surgeons would not purchase the laser as an individual, but some do. Depending on the volume of surgery they perform, they could charge $2,400 per eye and be losing money or barely breaking even. When the lasers were first approved, some surgeons thought laser vision correction would be the next gold rush. They ran out and bought lasers. As we discussed earlier, PRK did not deliver the initial volume of cases that is now being seen with LASIK. Fortunately, with the success of LASIK many of these centers have gone "in the black," but it has been a long, costly struggle.

Another option for obtaining the laser is for the doctor or clinic to lease it. Arrangements can be made to pay on a "per use" basis, however, minimum usage levels have to be met or the clinic must pay the difference on the lease.

More typically a surgeon gets access to a laser shared by a group of surgeons. This may be a group of doctors who come together to purchase or lease the laser or a hospital or surgery center that does so. Another means of access is through a corporate owned laser center. Back in the beginning of the "laser gold rush" in the U.S., several corporations sprang up with the intent of running laser centers around the country, hoping to profit from facility fees. More than one went bankrupt or sold out to a competing company. Again, the laser vision correction market was initially overestimated. The companies that remain are performing as much surgery in their centers as the busiest private clinics and surgery centers.

One creative approach is a mobile laser, which is transported from one office or surgery center to another on a truck. This laser is rolled in to the office and taken away at the end of the day or days. This is referred to as a "roll on, roll off" laser. The FDA required separate safety and result data for approval of the mobile laser. The laser is transported by a certified technician, who tests and calibrates it once he rolls it into the facility. This has enabled access to lasers in towns where full time use could not be supported or justified.

Fees for using the laser will vary depending on the setting described above and, more importantly, on the volume of cases performed at the facility. The more cases that are done, the lower the cost per case. The going rate for use of the laser, for LASIK, is $1,000 to $1,200 per eye, depending on the above variables. PRK is generally slightly less because the microkeratome and disposable blade are not necessary. You may be asked to pay the fee for use of the laser directly to the facility and write a separate check to the surgeon for his professional fee, or the fees may be bundled together in one charge.

Royalty Fees

In addition to the cost of purchasing or leasing a laser there is a $250 royalty fee charged every time the laser is used! A card similar to a credit card must be inserted to trigger the laser. One card for each treatment. Two cards for both eyes, even if they're done on the same day.

This fee is included in the $1,000 to $1,200 per eye estimated facility charge. If LASIK costs $2,000 to $2,500 per eye, the royalty fee is 10 to 12.5 percent of the total charge or 20 to 25 percent of the facility charge alone. The royalty fee is paid directly to the laser manufacturer. This is a large cost to the consumer and to the physicians providing the treatment. The laser manufacturers defend the fee on the basis of achieving a profitable return on the time and money invested in developing the technology.

VISX and Summit initially came together to form a partnership to collect royalty fees called Pillar Point. The Federal Trade Commission brought anti-trust charges. By avoiding competition with one another, there was no chance for the fees to be market driven. Despite the dissolution of Pillar Point, the laser companies still collect the same royalty fees. As more laser manufacturers receive FDA approval, perhaps these fees will come down as they try to compete with one another. This reduction could be passed on to the consumer.

Maintenance Fees

A third expense related to the laser is a service contract with the manufacturer. The cost is $52,000 a year. In addition, the argon and fluoride gases used to run the laser are paid for separately. These costs are part of the operating expenses of the laser facility. While they are not charged directly to the patient, they do raise the cost of providing surgery.

Microkeratome and Blade

The automated microkeratome costs about $50,000. Depending upon the number of cases that are performed, this expense raises the cost to the facility per case significantly. Regardless of volume, there is a charge for each disposable blade, which runs about $70. Once again, these expenses are paid by the facility and not charged additionally to the patient.

New technology requires new equipment. The Automatic Corneal Shaper, for example, does not make a large enough flap for the newly approved hyperopic treatment. The surgeon or the laser facility will have to buy a new $50,000 keratome to treat hyperopia.

Gaining Access to Patients

As noted in chapter seven, most patients in the age category for laser vision correction are under the care of optometrists for their glasses and contact lenses. "Vision plans," which cover routine exams for working people, are more often serviced by optometrists than ophthalmologists. Ophthalmology practices have typically positioned themselves to deal with the segment of the population that has eye problems, typically the elderly. So, most ophthalmology practices can't rely on the patients that come in to their offices for exams to generate enough patients to run a laser vision correction practice. Once a practice gets going, word of mouth referral helps bring in many patients. However, costs to gain access to additional patients are second only to use of the laser itself. These access costs include advertising, co-management fees and satellite offices.

Advertising

Costs of newspaper or radio advertisements announcing seminars or free screenings add up quickly. In small metropolitan areas a single 30-second radio commercial may cost $100 or less, but in major cities the cost may be $600 or more, depending on the popularity of the radio station. The commercial must be aired many times to announce the seminar effectively. Newspaper advertisements also vary in cost from hundreds to thousands of dollars for a single ad, depending on the city and the size of the ad. These advertising costs reduce the profit margin for the surgeon, and contribute to the overall expense of providing laser vision correction.

Co-Management Fees

In order to increase their access to laser vision correction patients, surgeons will sometimes work out arrangements with the primary eye doctor to provide your care following surgery, the "**post operative care**." The primary doctor needs to be specifically trained to do so."**Co-manage-ment**" eases the concerns of the optometrist about losing you to the laser surgeon, and enables him or her to actively participate in your care.

The surgeon reduces his charge to you since he is providing the surgery only, and the primary eye doctor charges for the post-operative care. Therefore, you do not pay any extra, but the surgeon makes less money for performing the same surgery.

Satellite or Separate Offices

As ophthalmologists enter the arena of laser vision correction, they may find that their offices are not located in an area that attracts younger patients. They may determine that opening a satellite office in another location may be more conducive to developing a refractive surgery practice. Costs include additional rent and leasehold improvements, eye examination equipment, office furniture and equipment, and personnel.

Some doctors are finding that even if the geographic location of the practice is good, the physical office layout is not. They may need to establish a separate waiting room and staff to service the laser patients.

Time Away From Established Practice

Time spent developing a laser vision correction practice is time away from the established ophthalmology practice, which is profitable. The former requires giving seminars, providing free screening exams, time spent traveling to the laser facility — which may not be close — and time to perform the lasers.

Patients are unlikely to think about or be concerned by the above. This information is given however, to help you understand why laser vision correction may not be as profitable as you might imagine.

Are Fees Likely to Come Down?

For all the reasons explained above, laser vision correction fees are not likely to change significantly in the next few years. New software and equipment will continue to drive up expenses, or at least prevent them from coming down. It can't be compared to home computers, where millions are sold each year. There's a limit to the number of half-million dollar lasers that can be sold.

Financing

How many of us can afford to walk into a car dealership and pay cash? Most laser surgeons offer a financing program, either through the local bank or a special credit company. This enables patients to make affordable payments, often as little as $100 a month. It becomes a matter of priorities for you. How much is a lifetime of vision correction worth? As much as a big screen TV? This is something that you will need to decide for yourself.

9
Training, Fellowships, Experience: What's it All About?

*W*e briefly described the training required of an ophthalmologist in chapter seven. As you recall an ophthalmologist attends college and medical school, then completes an internship in general medicine or surgery followed by a three year hospital-based residency in ophthalmology. For some, the road does not end there but continues on with a fellowship in a sub-specialty area. This might be retina, pediatrics, glaucoma, oculoplastics or corneal and refractive surgery. Fellowships are primarily intended for doctors who either seek an academic career at a university, teaching residents, or those who wish to work in a private practice primarily caring for patients with one of these specific problems.

In this chapter we will review the training involved in cornea and refractive surgery and some of the advertising claims you need to be able to sort through as an educated patient.

General Ophthalmology

Most ophthalmologists do not complete a fellowship but intead, directly enter private practice following their residency. They should be well prepared to handle most situations that arise and will refer patients with specific problems to a subspecialist. For most general ophthalmologists the primary surgical procedure performed is cataract surgery, the "bread and butter" of their practices.

The age of the ophthalmologist, and more specifically the years in which they served their residency, will determine whether they had any exposure to refractive surgery during their training. Most ophthalmologists gained their exposure to refractive surgery after their residency, as part of continuing education. Radial keratotomy or "RK," began in the late 1970s and was not taught in most residency programs. Excimer laser surgery was performed in small numbers in the early 1990s as part of clinical trials and gained FDA approval in 1995.

Cutting edge advances in refractive surgery arise in the private sector. From a historical perspective, it helps to understand that refractive surgery required a major change in the mindset of an ophthalmologist. As medical doctors we are trained to diagnose and treat disease — cataracts, glaucoma, crossed eyes, retinal detachment. When surgery is required to treat one of these disorders we recommend it to the patient and explain the risks and benefits. Recognizing that complications can arise in any surgery, it is easier for us to accept them when they occur in a diseased eye, one that was not functioning normally when it underwent surgery.

Refractive surgery was a major challenge to the profession of ophthalmology and stimulated heated controversy. Surgeons pursuing refractive surgery, initally RK, argued that their patients were not functioning normally, but were handicapped in their lifestyle by thick glasses and contact lenses. Others countered that it was not reasonable to expose these patients to any potential complications or loss of vision. The initial pioneers in RK were scorned by some of their colleagues.

As you might imagine, the first doctors to develop and refine radial keratotomy in the early 1980s were not university based ophthalmology professors. Refractive surgery was too hot politically for most corneal departments to handle. While there are a few exceptions, as a rule academic programs are conservative. That's a good approach in most circumstances; they wait until treatments are tried and proven before teaching them to their students.

Laser vision correction has put an end to the controversy. It is an accepted and approved treatment for refractive errors. Times certainly have changed.

Clinical Trials

While radial keratotomy began outside university centers, FDA clinical trials for laser vision correction often started there. The number of private practice physicians who initially could afford to get involved was limited by the great expense of obtaining a laser and the limited number of patients who could be treated. Some did, particularly in Canada where lesser government restrictions meant surgery could be performed in large numbers. The trial sites used initially are often used again for subsequent studies, in a self-perpetuating fashion.

Although the physicians involved in FDA clinical trials include some of the best refractive surgeons in the country, there are as many or more excellent LASIK and PRK surgeons who have not participated in them.

Corneal Fellowship

Following residency in ophthalmology, some physicians choose to complete an additional one to two years of study of the cornea and external diseases that affect the eye. External diseases refer to infections, allergic conditions and ocular surface problems. Hereditary disorders and abnormalities such as keratoconus are studied as well. Traditionally these programs provided additional training in corneal transplantation beyond that received in residency. A transplant is the replacement of a diseased cornea with a normal one taken from a donor eye.

For reasons discussed above, corneal fellowships were very slow to adopt and introduce refractive surgery into their curriculum. When I served my corneal fellowship in 1987, there were very few that did. I was fortunate that my fellowship at UCLA did have a refractive surgery clinic that was a vital part of the program. At the present time most corneal fellowship programs now include refractive surgery.

One important fact for the consumer is that not all corneal fellowships, in regard to refractive surgery, are created equal. However, they all provide much beneficial experience in recognizing abnormal corneas and patients who should not have laser vision correction. They teach how to perform surgery on the cornea, treat astigmatism, and manage normal and abnormal healing of the cornea. In summary, corneal fellowship provides a great foundation toward becoming an excellent corneal and refractive surgeon.

Training in Laser Vision Correction

How does a surgeon become trained in laser vision correction in 1999? The first part of the training is to attend a PRK training program, sponsored by the individual laser manufacturers. Thus, VISX Corporation sponsors a program taught by physicians, and Summit has its own course. The FDA specifies teaching requirements. These include several hours of lecture material and a wet lab, in which the surgeon is familiarized with the laser. Usually animal eyes obtained from meat processing plants are used for practice. Certification is withheld until the physician treats his first patient under the supervision of a **proctor**, an experienced laser surgeon.

Training in LASIK is less formalized. The most commonly used microkeratome is manufactured by Chiron, which requires a two day certificate course before it will sell microkeratome blades to the surgeon. As with the PRK course, a combination of lecture and wet lab is used. Videotapes of LASIK surgery are shown or live surgery is performed by an experienced surgeon. In the wet lab physicans practice the assembly, use, disassembly and maintainence of the microkeratome. Pig eyes are used to practice creating the corneal flap.

Additional Training:
Reducing the Learning Curve

Any additional education is at the discretion of the physician. The minimal training described above will not prepare beginning surgeons for all they will encounter when performing surgery on patients. The lack of experience of a novice surgeon can lead to a higher rate of surgical complications. This is referred to as the surgeon's **"learning curve."** Supplemental training should be pursued for the safety of the patient. The learning curve does not have to be steep, or riddled with complications. There are several ways that this can be accomplished.

Observing an experienced surgeon at his office and laser suite is a great help. This serves to reinforce concepts taught at the courses, and allows a one-on-one learning experience. Many surgeries can be observed, the preoperative evaluation of the patients reviewed and post-operative patients examined. This should be done with at least one mentor surgeon, for one or more days.

Additional practice making the keratectomy on pig eyes is also important. Using the microkeratome is a mechanical skill that can be rehearsed. However, placing the suction ring on a pig's eye mounted on a holder is much easier than on a real live human patient, where eyebrows, eyelids and lashes get in the way and challenge the surgeon. Getting the keratome on its track is also much more challenging.

Perhaps the most important step in securing excellent results in the beginning of a laser surgeon's practice is "proctoring." The presence of an experienced surgeon in the laser suite helps tremendously, particularly for the first several cases. One prominent malpractice company requires that the first five cases be proctored. In the best case scenario, the proctor may stand uselessly in the room. That's great. However, the performing surgeon may have questions that arise, even when things are going well, and it's reassuring for him to have immediate feedback.

Why Does Experience Matter?

Surgical experience improves the manual, technical skills required for LASIK. The single most challenging step of the procedure is to create the corneal flap. The eyelids are spread apart by a wire speculum. Some patients have easy, wide exposure and others have deep set, sunken eyes. Therefore, applying the suction ring may be easy or difficult. Other technical steps include:

- using the microkeratome to create the flap

- positioning the patient's head and monitoring his fixation during the treatment

- repositioning the flap and checking for proper alignment.

The next most important area where experience is a factor is the prediction of outcome. How much correction does the laser provide? It's not as simple as you might imagine. If the patient has 6 diopters of myopia, does the surgeon set the laser at 6 diopters, or 6 diopters less some adjustment or fudge factor? This varies with the laser brand (VISX or Summit) the individual laser and the surgeon (see below). Often 10 to 15 percent will be subtracted from the prescription to avoid overcorrection. The more procedures a surgeon does with the same laser, the more comfortable he will become in knowing what adjustment factor, if any, to apply.

Another experience-related issue involves fluid, which escapes from the corneal cells as they are being lasered. Fluid accumulates in the center of the cornea and can absorb the laser energy, causing the central cornea to receive less laser treatment than the periphery, where no moisture is produced. A few years ago this created a problem known as **"central islands"** for some PRK patients. Laser manufacturers addressed this complication by having the laser apply more treatment in the center than the periphery. However, some patients give off more fluid than others. During the ablation the surgeon must decide whether to stop one or more times to use a tiny cellulose sponge to wipe up the droplet. This can affect results. If there is a lot of moisture and the surgeon does not wipe, there may be an undercorrection—but if he wipes too much, he might get an overcorrection. Again, with experience the surgeon will learn how wiping affects his results and will adjust appropriately.

The third area in which experience plays an important role is the management and avoidance of complications. This includes recognizing before, during or after the procedure when something needs correction and knowing how to manage it. Good training helps to reduce the rate of complications by preventing them. Unfortunately, surgery doesn't always go perfectly, and even when it all goes well on the operating table, complications can still arise during the healing period. These were reviewed in Chapter 4. The more surgery a doctor performs, the more complications he will manage.

All the above being said, there are variables beyond the control of the surgeon. Individual variations in healing will affect the outcome of the procedure. When the results were quoted in chapter five, one of the reasons for failing to achieve 20/20 for more than 60 percent, is due to this factor. Research continues for drugs that can help modify the healing response. Also, reliance on machinery — computer driven lasers and microkeratomes — no matter how sophisticated, is another potential source of problems.

Proper management of complications is key to damage control. Experience makes a difference. Having a proctor in the laser room will help if a problem arises during the procedure, and consultation with an experienced surgeon can help in the successful management of a problem that arises in the post-operative period. In this era of the Internet, laser surgeons can now interact around the world. This helps identify problems that occur infrequently and lets surgeons benefit from the experience of others.

What About General Ophthalmology Experience?

How much benefit does a beginning LASIK surgeon get from his years of experience in performing eye surgery other than laser vision correction? Usually, we are referring to cataract surgery and laser procedures for glaucoma and retinal diseases.

The microsurgical skills required for performing these procedures do overlap with LASIK to a degree and are essential for becoming an expert at the latter. However, they are no substitute for actual experience with LASIK as described above. In cataract surgery the doctor uses delicate instruments in both hands, while sitting and viewing the patient's eye through a microscope. The surgeon's feet are positioned on two footpedals, one to work the focus of the microscope and the other to manipulate the machine that removes the cataract. These same skills are used in LASIK plus additional ones that must be mastered.

Deceptive Advertising

Related to the issue of experience in general eye surgery is a concern about deceptive advertising. When an eye surgeon does not have much experience performing PRK or LASIK, he will sometimes try to boast about having performed large numbers of eye surgeries or laser surgeries. He will not specify in advertisements that the eye surgeries performed were cataracts and the lasers were for glaucoma or retina treatments—not PRK or LASIK. This is quite misleading to the patient. You may have to specifically question the doctor on how many LASIK procedures he has performed to ascertain his experience.

Honesty Is the Best Policy

If the doctor is wise, he will be truthful. It's hard to get a laser vision correction practice started. It takes word of mouth referrals among patients, and when a doctor has done none, or just a few, that's slow to happen. No surgeon wants to lose you to another, and it's embarrasing to admit his inexperience. However, it's better for the surgeon to be straight with you and explain that he is just getting started. I told patients, in the beginning, exactly that. I reviewed my prior refractive surgery experience with RK and keratomileusis, and my laser vision correction training to date. I also arranged for an experienced proctor to be in the laser room, and the patient was made aware of this as well. Limited experience does not equate with inferior results. As an example, the first LASIK patient that I operated on (-6.75 diopters) achieved 20/20 vision in both eyes without glasses!

What Makes a Great Refractive Surgeon?

Hopefully, after reading this book you will have a better appreciation for everything the surgeon does in achieving an excellent result with laser vision correction surgery. In counseling patients who are interested in the procedures, surgeons have a tendency to underplay the seriousness, the multiplicity of events that must come together for a perfect result. This is understandable. They don't want to scare you away.

This approach is not necessary and undermines your appreciation for what you are having done. You should understand the complexity of the procedure. Though the statistics speak for the success of the procedure, there are complications that can get in the way of your intended excellent result.

Laser vision correction cannot be just another procedure added to the menu of surgery performed in a general ophthalmology practice. It takes a committment of time and resources to learn a whole new set of skills and develop a new type of surgical practice, different from a senior citizen cataract practice. LASIK must be performed regularly, not done here and there for the occasional patient who walks in and expresses interest. Thus, the first step toward being a great refractive surgeon takes place in the heart of the individual.

Let's assemble the components in the path toward excellence. First, we need a well trained ophthalmologist with years of experience spent in developing the fine motor skills to perform eye surgery through a microscope. Preferably, he's had years of experience with refractive surgery. The surgeon needs to be well trained in laser vision correction, as described above. This includes certification courses and hopefully additional time out of his practice to study with experienced surgeons.

Next, the surgeon and his staff needs to spend a good amount of time with you before surgery. This should include a careful measurement of your refractive error. It does not matter how good the laser is: if the information isn't accurate, it's not worth a dime. He needs to understand why you desire laser surgery and then to help you understand the risks and benefits so that you can make an informed decision. Your eye must be carefully examined for any conditions that could lead to a bad result, such as keratoconus, and your medical history needs to be screened as well.

The surgeon needs to be experienced with the specific laser that is to be used, or to confer with other surgeons who are using this particular laser. The temperature and humidity of the laser room are also factors. He needs to know how close the laser comes to making the entered correction. The surgeon will use this information to adjust your correction. It's not as simple as pressing a button.

On the day of surgery, the laser will be calibrated by a technician, and the surgeon must verify that it is to his satisfaction. Additional testing plates are available to check for the homogeneity of the beam (see pg 108-109). The laser can go out of calibration between cases on a given day.

Only now do we come to the critical steps involved in creating the corneal flap. For starters, the microkeratome must be assembled by the surgeon or a technician under the supervision of the surgeon. Its proper function must be verified in a test run. The blade must be carefully handled from the moment it leaves the package. Any small damage to the cutting edge can ruin the flap. The microkeratome needs to be watched to be certain the blade doesn't contact any other instruments while awaiting use.

Next comes the surgical skills discussed earlier in creating the corneal flap, the critical step of LASIK. A trained eye monitors your fixation as you stare at the light and skilled hands guide the repositioning of the flap, making sure the alignment in the bed is perfect. Finally, the surgeon's experienced eyes watch yours as you heal, alert for any deviations from the course required for your improved eyesight without glasses.

Congratulations! You're on your way to a whole new life. If you're as thrilled as I think you will be, take a moment to let your surgeon know. That's the joy that makes this all worthwhile for us.

GLOSSARY

Accommodation: the process by which the focus of a person's eye changes from a distant object to one that is closer, as for reading. The internal crystalline lens of the eye changes its shape to *accommodate*. As we get older, our ability to *accommodate* decreases and reading glasses are necessary. See also presbyopia and cycloplegia.

AK (Astigmatic Keratotomy): an incision, using a diamond knife, made in the cornea to correct astigmatism. The incision is made in the steep axis of the astigmatism, causing the cornea to flatten.

Aphakia: describes an eye which has no crystalline lens. A patient whose crystalline lens has been removed due to a cataract or trauma and who has not received a plastic replacement lens, or intraocular lens, is aphakic. With the development of intraocular lenses, patients are no longer left aphakic following cataract surgery. Aphakic patients require thick "cataract glasses" or contact lenses to see.

Aqueous humor: the salty fluid produced inside the eye that creates an internal eye pressure. See intraocular pressure and glaucoma.

Astigmatism: a common condition in which the cornea is oval-shaped, like a football—not round, like a baseball. Along one axis, the cornea is more steeply curved and has a shorter radius of curvature; along the other axis, the cornea has a flatter curve and a longer radius of curvature. See axes.

Axes: the axis, or direction, of a patient's astigmatism is measured in degrees, from zero to one hundred eighty degrees. Ninety degrees is vertical, and one hundred eighty degrees is horizontal. These two axes are usually perpendicular to each other, one horizontal and one vertical.

Bandage contact lens: a soft contact lens used for comfort while the surface of the cornea heals from a corneal abrasion or PRK laser surgery.

Best Corrected Visual Acuity: a measurement of how well a person can see with the best measurable prescription for glasses or contact lenses. See visual acuity.

Bilateral surgery: surgery in which both eyes of a patient are operated on during the same session. First one eye is treated, then the other.

Broad beam laser: an excimer laser that delivers a beam with a six millimeter diameter.

Cataract: a cloudiness of the crystalline lens that is common with aging.

Central island: a complication of laser vision correction in which the center of the cornea receives less treatment than the surrounding tissue, leaving the patient undercorrected. It now occurs less frequently due to an improvement in the laser software that allows more treatment to the center of the cornea.

Cold spot: an area of reduced energy output in the laser beam. A cold spot does not remove as much corneal tissue as needed, resulting in an undercorrection. This is more of a problem with broad beam lasers than scanning lasers.

Co-management: treatment in which the primary eye doctor, often an optometrist, provides most of the post-operative care of the patient, instead of the laser surgeon.

Contraindications: existent conditions that preclude the use of a specific medication or surgical treatment on a patient.

Cornea: the clear, outer window to the eye on which a patient places his contact lens. The cornea is arranged in layers of collagen, or lamellae, stacked perpendicular to one another.

Corneal abrasion: an injury that rubs off the epithelium, the outermost layer of the cornea. Corneal abrasions heal in one to five days. Also known as a "scratched" cornea.

Corneal ring segments: see intrastromal corneal ring segments.

Corneal topography (corneal mapping): a map of the surface of the cornea that reveals astigmatism and other abnormalities. A series of concentric circles is projected onto the cornea, and a computer measures the curvature along each ring. A colored map is generated from this information to detect those abnormal corneas for which laser vision correction is not indicated.

Corneal transplant (penetrating keratoplasty): replacement of the central portion of an abnormal cornea with tissue from a donor.

Corneal ulcer: an infection of the cornea. Corneal ulcers can occur because of contact lens use or laser vision correction. Though infrequent, corneal ulcers are more likely to occur with PRK than with LASIK.

Crystalline lens: the clear lens inside the eye that has an adjustable focus. With age, this lens may become clouded, a condition known as a cataract.

Cycloplegic agents: commonly called "dilating drops," cycloplegic agents act inside the eye to temporarily paralyze the muscle that focuses the crystalline lens, thereby blocking accommodation. Cycloplegic drugs cause the patient's pupils to dilate and blur his vision, making reading difficult.

Cycloplegic refraction: the measurement of an eyeglass prescription after the application of a cycloplegic agent. This allows a true determination of refractive error, ignoring error induced by the patient focusing his eye or accommodating.

Dilating drops: see cycloplegic agents.

Diopter: the standard unit of measurement of the amount of refractive error or strength of corrective eyeglasses and contact lenses. A "one diopter lens" is one that can converge parallel rays of light, in focus, one meter behind the lens.

Emmetropic: the absence of any refractive error, making eyeglasses or contact lenses unnecessary to see perfectly.

Endothelial cells: cells that line the inner surface of the cornea. The salty aqueous fluid of the eye comes in direct contact with the endothelial cell layer which must pump the fluid out of the cornea to keep it from swelling and the vision from becoming cloudy.

Endothelial cells do not multiply; once lost, they cannot be replaced except by transplant of donor tissue.

Excimer laser: the type of laser used to perform LASIK and PRK.

Eye Tracker: available in some lasers, it allows the laser to move in synchronization with the patient's eye during laser vision correction.

Farsighted: describes a person who sees distant objects well, but has trouble seeing close objects. The technical name of farsightedness is *hyperopia*.

Flap and zap: an expression used to describe the LASIK procedure. A superficial flap of the cornea is raised and the excimer laser is used to treat the underlying tissue. The flap is then repositioned without the need for sutures.

Fluence: the energy level of the laser beam used for LASIK and PRK. The fluence is checked to verify satisfactory output prior to the laser procedure.

Free cap: a complication of the LASIK procedure. A free cap of corneal tissue is removed and not left attached by a hinge. The cap is realigned to marks that are made at the beginning of surgery. Creating a free cap is not a serious problem. LASIK was initially performed by deliberately creating a free cap; leaving a hinge was developed later.

Fuch's Corneal Dystrophy: a hereditary condition characterized by a diminished number of endothelial cells. With age, there is continued attrition of these cells. Eventually, a critical level may be reached in which the cornea swells and vision becomes blurred. Ultimately, patients with Fuch's Corneal Dystrophy may require a cornea transplant if vision blurs significantly.

Glaucoma: damage to the optic nerve by elevated fluid pressure within the eye. Glaucoma can be treated with eyedrops, lasers, or surgery that reduces the amount of fluid, and relieves "intraocular pressure."

Haze: a clouding of the cornea following excimer laser treatment that is primarily a complication of PRK. Haze is treated with topical cortisone eye drops. If it is severe enough, haze may reduce vision until it clears. Patients with haze often are undercorrected, sometimes necessitating additional laser treatment.

Herpes: a group of viruses that afflict man. Herpes simplex, Type I, causes cold sores and may produce a recurrent infection of the eye. Repeated attacks may cause scarring and reduced vision. Herpes infections never leave the body, but lay dormant instead. Under certain conditions, such as exposure to sunlight, stress, the common cold and use of topical steroid eyedrops, the virus may flare.

Herpes keratitis: a corneal infection caused by Herpes virus, Type I.

High myopia: usually defined as more than six diopters of myopia. Patients with high myopia are more prone to develop retinal detachment even without having any laser surgery.

Homogeneity: a laser beam having uniform energy across its diameter.

Hot spots: a laser beam having one or more spots of increased energy relative to the remainder of the beam. A lack of desired homogeneity.

Hyperope: a person with hyperopia.

Hyperopia: an eye with a short axial length and a cornea and crystalline lens too weak to bring an image to focus on the retina. The technical term for "farsightedness."

Hyperopic shift: a change in a patient's eyeglass prescription in which the person becomes more hyperopic, or farsighted, than they were initially. This was a significant problem with radial keratotomy surgery, in which long-term results showed a continued hyperopic shift in many patients. This has not been a problem with PRK and LASIK.

Intrastromal Corneal Ring Segments (ICRS): small, curved, plastic rings surgically positioned in the peripheral cornea that flatten the central cornea to correct myopia. Presently approved for use in the United States for correction of myopia up to three diopters only. No correction is yet available for astigmatism or hyperopia.

Incisional refractive surgery: any surgical procedure performed with a diamond microsurgical knife to make incisions in the cornea to reduce or eliminate the need for eyeglasses and contact lenses. Primarily refers to radial keratotomy (RK) and astigmatic keratotomy (AK), procedures that have largely been replaced by laser vision correction.

Intraocular lens (IOL): a small, plastic lens, about 1/4 inch in diameter, that is inserted into the eye to allow it to focus. Intraocular lenses have been used for decades to correct vision following cataract surgery. Clinical trials are underway in younger patients (who do not have cataracts) using similar lenses placed in front of the crystalline lens to reduce or eliminate the need for eyeglasses.

Intraocular pressure: the fluid pressure inside the eye determined by the balance between the amount of aqueous fluid produced and the amount drained. If the drain becomes clogged with age, the fluid pressure can rise above normal levels, causing glaucoma. Elevated intraocular pressure cannot be felt by the patient, however.

IOP: intraocular pressure

Iridectomy: a surgical incision made in the iris, the colored part of the eye, to relieve a buildup of intraocular pressure caused by a physical obstruction of the internal drain of the eye. This procedure is unnecessary for the vast majority of patients who have glaucoma.

Irregular astigmatism: a corneal surface that is not smooth, creating blurred vision that is not correctable by eyeglasses. However, gas-permeable contact lenses may correct this problem by providing a smooth, round surface to focus light.

Keratectomy: to incise or excise a portion of the cornea.

Keratoconus: an abnormal cornea that assumes the shape of a cone instead of a sphere. Keratoconus is associated with reduced visual acuity that initially can be corrected by the smooth surface of a gas-permeable contact lens. As the condition progresses, however, a cornea transplant may be necessary to correct vision.

Laser: an instrument that uses energy from light to cut or burn tissue. Lasers differ in the wavelength of light used to generate the laser beam.

Laser Vision Correction: use of an excimer laser to correct nearsightedness, farsightedness, and astigmatism. Two procedures, LASIK and PRK, are used to accomplish this.

LASIK (laser-assisted keratomileusis in situ, "flap and zap"): a procedure in which a special instrument, the microkeratome, cuts a thin flap of corneal tissue. The excimer laser is then used to reshape the cornea beneath the flap. After reshaping, the flap is repositioned without sutures. Visual recovery and healing is quick.

Learning curve: the learning process experienced by a surgeon performing initial cases of a new surgical technique. Procedures that are difficult to master or that have a high rate of complications have a "steep" learning curve.

Lenticular astigmatism: astigmatism caused by an uneven surface of the crystalline lens of the eye. Most astigmatism derives more from the cornea than the lens.

Loss of best spectacle corrected visual acuity: a patient who can see better with eyeglasses *before* surgery than *after* surgery has suffered a loss of best spectacle corrected visual acuity.

Low myopia: up to three diopters of myopia.

Manifest refraction: a determination of a person's eyeglass prescription made by asking that person to subjectively choose between different lenses. Most eyeglass wearers are familiar with the process as the dreaded procedure in which they are asked "Which is clearer—lens number one, or lens number two?"

M.D.: a medical doctor. A graduate of medical school. The eye care M.D. is the ophthalmologist, who is trained to perform eye surgery as well as manage medical problems of the eye.

Microkeratome: a machine that creates the corneal flap for LASIK. Most use a disposable metal blade that oscillates at an extremely high rate to cut a smooth flap.

Moderate myopia: three to six diopters of myopia.

Monovision: using one eye for reading and one for distance viewing. This is generally accomplished with contact lenses, fitting one for near and one for far. Monovision can be created with laser vision correction. As an example, one eye of a myope can be treated for distance, and the other eye left untreated, or only partially treated, to allow reading vision without glasses.

Myope: a person with myopia.

Myopia: a condition caused by an eye that has grown too long in its axial length, causing images to focus in front of the retina, instead of directly on it. Myopia is often called "nearsightedness," since a myope can usually read without eyeglasses.

Nearsighted: a synonym for myopia.

Nomogram: a table created by analyzing post-operative results to determine an adjustment factor to apply to a patient's prescription for laser vision correction. As an example, when the results of 5 diopter myopes (aged forty-five) are examined, it might be determined that 10 percent should be subtracted from the five diopter prescription to yield a perfect zero correction result. In this case, the laser would be set to treat 4.50 diopters.

Age, gender, humidity and altitude of the laser room, and the amount of myopia all affect the outcome of the surgery and the adjustment factor used for laser vision correction.

O.D.: 1. Doctor of Optometry. An optometrist. One of two groups of eye doctors. 2. ocular dexter, the right eye.

Ocular dexter: the right eye.

Ophthalmologist: a medical doctor (M.D.) who specializes in treating medical and surgical eye problems and performs LASIK surgery. One of two groups of eye doctors.

O.S.: the abbreviation for ocular sinister, the left eye.

Ocular sinister: the left eye.

Optical zone: the diameter, in millimeters, of the center of the cornea that is treated by the laser in LASIK and PRK. If an imaginary circle were drawn around a patient's pupil outlining the area that is to be treated by the laser, the diameter of that circle would be the optical zone. Larger optical zones provide better night vision since our pupils dilate at night.

Orthokeratology: a non-surgical procedure to lessen myopia by deliberately fitting a hard contact lens too tight in order to flatten the cornea. Unfortunately, results are not permanent and only small changes in myopia can be induced. Laser vision correction provides a far superior option.

Overcorrection: to obtain more correction with the laser than intended. When treating myopia, an overcorrection results in the patient becoming hyperopic. A retreatment can be performed for hyperopia to bring the patient closer to the intended result.

Phakic intraocular lens (phakic IOL): a small, plastic lens surgically implanted in the eye to correct myopia or hyperopia in patients who still have their crystalline lens in place, i.e., in patients who are too young to have cataracts.

Phakic: an eye that has a crystalline lens to focus images and has not yet undergone cataract surgery.

Photoablation: the use of laser light energy to excise tissue.

PRK (photorefractive keratectomy): the initial procedure used for laser vision correction. The epithelium covering the cornea is wiped off, then the laser is used to reshape the cornea. Several days are required for the surface of the cornea to heal and visual recovery is much slower than LASIK. However, long-term results are equal.

Post Operative Care: management of the patient after surgery. For LASIK, the patient is typically seen at one day, one week, and one, three, and six months after surgery. These visits can be performed by the laser surgeon or by a trained primary eye doctor.

Presbyopia: a need for reading glasses that develops after age forty. Presbyopia develops because of the loss of accommodation that occurs with age.

Proctor: an experienced laser eye surgeon who observes and/or makes suggestions to a novice surgeon during his initial procedures.

Pseudophakic (pseudo: false; phakic: lens): an eye that has undergone cataract surgery and replacement of the crystalline lens by a plastic intraocular lens.

Pupillary Block Glaucoma: an abnormally high pressure in the eye caused by a physical obstruction of the pupil by an intraocular lens.

Radial Keratotomy (RK): a procedure to correct myopia that uses 4 or 8 slit-like incisions in the cornea to flatten its curvature. Radial keratotomy was popular before the advent of laser vision correction procedures.

Refractive error: any condition that requires glasses or contact lenses to see clearly. There are four types of refractive errors: myopia (or nearsightedness), hyperopia (or farsightedness), astigmatism and presbyopia.

Refractive surgery: any surgical procedure for reducing or eliminating a refractive error. Includes RK, PRK, LASIK, phakic intraocular lenses, corneal rings, etc.

Regression: the loss of effect from a refractive surgical procedure. This is common and is expected during the early healing phase of laser vision correction. The laser's setting are made by taking into account an expected partial regression.

Regular astigmatism: a cornea that is shaped like a football (oval) instead of a baseball (round). The astigmatism is described by the two axes, or directions, in which the curvature is unequal. In regular astigmatism, the two axes are at ninety degrees, perpendicular to one another.

Retreatment: a second laser treatment for PRK or LASIK performed to provide additional treatment for an eye that was undercorrected or overcorrected by the initial surgery. With LASIK, the original corneal flap can be surgically lifted, or a new flap can be cut, leaving the original flap healed in place.

RK: see radial keratotomy.

Sands of the Sahara (diffuse interlamellar keratitis): a complication of LASIK having unknown etiology. Believed to be an allergic reaction that results in a non-infectious infiltrate, causing hazy vision that clears with steroid eye drops.

Scanning laser: a newer excimer laser having technology that uses a small beam one to two millimeters in diameter. The smaller beam is rotated by mirrors to treat the full six millimeter optical zone. In comparison, broad beam lasers have a six millimeter beam that treats the whole optical zone at one time.

Striae: folds in the corneal cap, a complication of LASIK. Striae are corrected by lifting the corneal flap and repositioning it.

Twenty-twenty (20/20): the ideal, normal visual acuity. The person being tested can see letters from twenty feet away that an ideal, normal person can also see from the same distance.

Uncorrected visual acuity: how well a person can see without eyeglasses or contact lenses. Also called unaided visual acuity.

Undercorrection: less than a full correction of a patient's refractive error. Can be managed by applying more laser treatment at a later date.

Visual acuity: a measurement of how well a person can see, determined by a patient reading an eye chart. A large "E" is on the top line of the chart, and progressively smaller letters follow below. The worse a person's vision, the larger the denominator of the fraction that describes his visual acuity. Thus, 20/400 vision is poor, 20/20 vision is excellent. If you wish to drive a car without glasses, the legal requirement is 20/40 visual acuity.

INDEX

About the Author

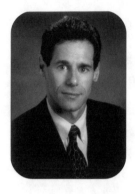

Matthew I. Ehrlich, M.D. is the founder of the Ehrlich Eye Center. He obtained his bachelor's degree at Union College in Schenectady, N.Y. and his medical degree at Albany Medical College in N.Y. in 1983. Both degrees were obtained in an accelerated six-year combined program. He was honored with memberships in Phi Beta Kappa and Alpha Omega Alpha.

His post graduate medical education began in the internal medicine department at Mt. Zion Hospital, University of California, San Francisco. He then served his residency in ophthalmology at Wills Eye Hospital in Philadelphia. In 1988 he completed his Cornea/Refractive Surgery Fellowship at the Jules Stein Eye Institute, University of California, Los Angeles (UCLA).

Dr. Ehrlich is board certified by the American Board of Ophthalmology and is a member of the American Medical Association, the American Academy of Ophthalmology, the American Society of Cataract and Refractive Surgery, the American College of Sports Medicine and the Sarasota County Medical Society. He has been practicing in the Sarasota, Florida area since 1988.

Dr. Ehrlich has lectured at major ophthalmology meetings and has appeared on television as both an expert guest and show host. He also has been a published medical author since 1981.

Dr. Ehrlich can be reached to schedule speaking engagements or interviews at (941) 371-8100, or on the internet sites: www.drehrlich.com & www.lasikbook.com

ORDER FORM

☎ **Telephone orders:** Call toll-free: **1-877-988-2020**
(Have your Visa or MasterCard ready).

▭ **Fax orders: 1-941-483-4240**

▭ **Online orders: www.lasikbook.com**

▭ **Mail orders: Doctors Advice Press**
217 The Esplanade South
Venice, Fl 34285

	Quantity	Amount
How to See Like A Hawk (BOOK) **$14.95**	_____	_____
The *LASIK Surgery Video* **$6.95** (Live surgery, Approx.7 min.)	_____	_____
Book and Video **$19.95**	_____	_____
Priority Shipping & Handling $4.00 first book or video ($2.00 each additional)		_____
Florida addresses add 7% sales tax		_____
Total Amount enclosed (U.S. funds)		_____

Company Name_____

Name_____

Address_____

City_____State_____ZIP_____

Telephone (____)_____

Payment:
  ☐ **Check** ☐ **MasterCard** ☐ **Visa**

Card number:_____Exp. date:_____

Name on card:_____